Perfect Calorie Counting

Kate Santon is a freelance writer and editor who specialises in food and drink. A firm believer in healthy dieting, she is the author of *Need to Know GI and GL Diets*, *Need to Know Calorie Counting*, and Collins' Gem guides on *GL Diets*, *Cholesterol* and *Fat-Burning Diets*.

Other titles in the *Perfect* Series

Perfect
Calorie Counting

Kate Santon

BOOKS

Published by Random House Books 2008

2 4 6 8 10 9 7 5 3 1

Copyright © Grapevine Publishing Services 2008
Calorie values are from *The Composition of Foods*, Food Standards Agency.
© Crown copyright material is reproduced with the permission of
the Controller of HMSO and Queen's Printer for Scotland.

Kate Santon has asserted her right under the Copyright, Designs
and Patents Act 1988 to be identified as the author of this work

First published in the United Kingdom in 2008 by
Random House Books

Random House Books
Random House, 20 Vauxhall Bridge Road,
London SW1V 2SA

www.randomhouse.co.uk

Addresses for companies within The Random House Group Limited
can be found at: www.randomhouse.co.uk/offices.htm

The Random House Group Limited Reg. No. 954009

A CIP catalogue record for this book
is available from the British Library

ISBN 9781847945181

The Random House Group Limited makes every effort to ensure that the
papers used in its books are made from trees that have been legally sourced
from well-managed and credibly certified forests. Our paper procurement
policy can be found at: www.randomhouse.co.uk/paper.htm

Printed and bound in the UK by CPI Bookmarque, Croydon, Surrey CR0 4TD

Contents

Introduction

Another day, another diet – or so it often seems. There are thousands of different diets out there, ranging from the apparently sensible to the obviously insane. Many encourage dieters to eliminate whole categories of food or buy particular products, and they sometimes state that 'calories don't count'. But they do. They always do.

Calories are just a measure of energy. Basically, if we take in more energy than our bodies use, we put weight on; if we use more than we take in, the weight comes off. It is a more complex relationship than that brief statement implies when you go into it in detail, but this is the essence of all diets. Those diets which assure people that 'calories don't matter' work – when they work at all – by restricting the calories consumed, despite what they state.

Unfortunately many, especially the freaky, faddy diets (and they are usually the ones that make this claim) can actually harm dieters' health instead of improving it. In addition, any success gained is almost always wiped out when people stop following the diets and return to their previous patterns of eating. Finally, the restrictions and substitutions of these diets don't help most of us, who need to lose weight because we like food.

In recent years, some much healthier diets have been developed. These encourage healthy eating and lifestyle change, both of which are necessary for the best results and for keeping the weight off in the long term. They also offer much more freedom. The GI and GL diets are almost unique in having been generally welcomed by the medical establishment, but they do have one disadvantage – it can be easy to eat too much.

This is where the modern approach to calorie counting comes in. The old form of calorie counting – effectively eating whatever you wanted as long as you kept to below a certain number of calories, and adding everything up obsessively – did work, but didn't encourage the lifestyle change needed to make a permanent difference. Dieters could consume their 1,500 calories per day entirely in beer or sweets, and that was fine as long as they lost weight. But it isn't really, and we all know it; we also know – probably through direct experience – that any weight lost on such a regime will come straight back. Yes, calorie counting does bring freedom, but with freedom comes responsibility.

A more modern attitude is to keep an eye on calories and eat a healthy, balanced diet, making some easy but radical changes which will help and then sticking to them. The only way to lose weight permanently is to control and balance your calories while eating healthily, but it's a lot less painful than it sounds. It does not have to take over your life, but it's not a quick fix – quick fixes don't help with long-term weight loss. You are in control though: you don't need to restrict whole groups of foods, you don't need to buy any strange powdered drinks or tubs of algae, you can still enjoy your meals, you can eat out and go to parties. It does need a bit of discipline and structure, and some willpower – there really is no such thing as a free lunch, in any sense – but there are many eating habits that can be adopted very easily, and they will soon become automatic.

Motivation is vital, so always remember that the aim of weight loss isn't just looking better, but being healthier too. In the long run, that's more important – and the benefits can be enormous.

1 How calorie counting works

The first thing to realise before you begin counting calories is that it can be simple. It doesn't have to dominate your life and you don't have to eat lots of weird and wonderful foods, though you do have to make some adjustments. Let's look at the basics of calorie counting; it is always easier to put something that could require fundamental changes into practice when you understand roughly how it works.

Dieting by counting calories is essentially logical and straightforward. It uses the relationship between the energy we take in as food and the energy our bodies use to function, as do most weight-loss programmes in some form or other. The advantage – one advantage – of calorie counting is that the relationship is obvious. By itself, however, it won't work; you need to combine it with eating healthily.

Basically, when you consistently consume more calories than your body uses, you put weight on because the excess energy is stored in the form of fat. If you use more energy than you get from the food you eat, the extra comes from the stored fat and the weight drops off. So, if energy in is greater than energy out, your weight goes up; if energy out is greater than energy in, your weight goes down. But there's more to it than that; you need to eat healthily as well.

Life is impossible without food because it provides both necessary energy and vital nutrients; if you don't get enough of those you could be damaging your health. Nutrients are the chemical building blocks the body requires in order to grow and develop normally, manufacture hormones and DNA, build and repair cell walls, protect itself from damage … and perform many, many other functions. The energy itself comes from food as it is metabolised (changed into a form that the body can use).

What is a calorie?

When food is metabolised it produces heat, and that heat is measured in kilocalories. To find out how many calories a food provides, scientists burn a weighed portion of it in a piece of equipment called a bomb calorimeter, along with a measured amount of cold water. As the food burns, the temperature of the water rises. Technically speaking, a kilocalorie is the amount of energy needed to raise the temperature of the water by one degree centigrade at sea level.

An individual calorie is one thousandth of a kilocalorie, as that name suggests. But a single calorie is a minute amount of energy, and the term 'calorie' has come to be generally used to mean a kilocalorie. Scientists and nutritionists use the more correct word 'kilocalorie', which is why its abbreviation – kCal – is seen on packaging. In this book, as in most other circumstances, calorie is used instead. 'Kilojoule' is another term that you may come across; again it appears on packaging, where it is shown as 'kJ'. Joules are the standard international units for measuring energy; the kilojoule is scientifically more accurate and internationally recognised, and is beginning to replace kilocalorie or calorie in some places. There are about 4.18 kilojoules to a kilocalorie, which is why labels might say something like '52 kCal/218 kJ'. In practice, though, the word 'calorie' is still in general use and is likely to remain so for some time.

One more thing. It is sometimes said that there are different types of calories, particularly 'carb calories' and 'fat calories'. These are not imaginary, but can effectively be ignored by most of us; they come from studies done under extremely unusual circumstances, when the body functions slightly differently. All food contains calories and all calories are basically the same; they all give you energy regardless of where they come from. So 1,500 calories of energy from wine, 1,500 calories from cabbage, 1,500 calories from fruit salad and 1,500 from chocolate are all basically identical. Calories are often assumed to be a measure of fat, but they are not. They are simply a measure of available energy; the difference comes in the nutritional benefits (or lack of) that the specific food contains, in the effect it has on your digestive system and, of course, in the effect it has on your health.

So, at the end of all that, if a pot of yoghurt has 78 calories, then eating it will make 78 calories of energy available to your body, which will then use what it needs and store the excess as fat. Every body does this differently; some people seem to store more energy more easily as fat than others.

The hormone insulin, which most of us link with diabetes, is associated with fat storage, and regulating the levels of insulin in the blood will help with weight loss. It is much easier for your body to keep insulin levels low and steady if you have a healthy diet, and some types of food are more helpful than others in this context.

Successful calorie counting isn't just a matter of totting up calories and keeping them low. You have to stay well at the same time, and preferably improve your health, and then there's the other half of the equation: energy out, or how your body uses energy. There are three basic ways, and understanding them helps you to set realistic targets as well as – hopefully – increase your weight loss.

Energy out - staying alive: the BMR

The basic energy you need to stay alive is the most significant of the three. Your body uses energy all the time, not just when you are moving about or exercising, but even when you are fast asleep or resting. Your heart is beating, blood is circulating around your body, your brain is sending instructions and receiving information, and you are breathing. You are barely aware of all these functions, but they use calories. In fact, these involuntary processes and the many others like them – every single cell in your body needs some energy – use most of the calories you take in (about 65–75 per cent, or even more). Your body needs this amount of energy just to keep its automatic functions running.

The rate at which you use this energy has several different names with slightly different interpretations: your resting energy expenditure, your resting metabolic rate (RMR, possibly the clearest name but not the most scientific of the measures) or your basal metabolic rate (BMR).

Because most calories are used in keeping the body going, your BMR is an important element in determining how much you weigh.

Basal metabolic rates are very variable; no two people's are the same. Sometimes your body just needs more energy – when you are pregnant, breastfeeding, or recovering from an operation, for instance. There's a genetic element in determining BMR, but that is far from being the whole story. There are some generalisations, though, based on age, sex and weight. Children have much higher metabolic rates than older people because they are growing; men have higher rates than women and fatter people have higher rates than thin people. That's right: it's not the other way round. A lot of people think that someone who is overweight 'just has a slow metabolism', that he or she burns calories more gradually than a slimmer person, but the opposite is true. The bigger the person, the higher their metabolic rate. It simply takes more energy to keep a larger body going, even when it's at rest.

There are other variations as well. Many women will have noticed that their appetite varies during their menstrual cycle, but it's not just appetite – it's a change in the BMR. The menopause can also affect it. Muscle comes into play, too. It uses more energy than fat, even at rest: more than 120 calories a day, where fat uses only 20. This is why men, who generally have more muscle than most women, have higher metabolic rates and can eat more without gaining weight – and that's why men and women have different calorie requirements. Men just need more energy to run their bodies, and because of that a man can eat more than a similarly sized woman without it affecting his weight in the same way.

Hormones – substances secreted by glands in the body – can have a profound impact. The sex hormones oestrogen, progesterone and testosterone prompt the development of things like distinctive male or female body shape and the presence of body hair when you hit puberty, but other hormones can affect your BMR in ways unrelated to your sex. Insulin is a hormone, secreted by the pancreas, and adrenaline is another, probably one of the best known. Adrenaline is released by the adrenal glands if you are excited or scared, and it boosts your BMR to produce the 'fight or flight' response – your heart beats you breathe more quickly, your muscles prepare for action and your digestive metabolism steps up a gear, converting food into energy at greater speed. The effects of adrenaline on your BMR are temporary, though, and it soon returns to a normal level.

The hormone thyroxin, which comes from the thyroid gland, can also affect your BMR. If you have hypothyroidism, the thyroid doesn't secrete enough thyroxin and your basal metabolic rate drops; if you have hyperthyroidism, it's the other way round. If you are finding it very difficult to lose weight despite serious, sensible attempts to do so, there is a chance that you might have an underactive thyroid. It may be worth while getting your doctor to check this out; it only involves a simple blood test and any problems can be treated very effectively.

There are a couple of other factors that can have an impact on your BMR. The first affects everyone: BMR declines with age. One of the reasons is that you slow down and your muscle mass tends to diminish, but that doesn't mean that BMR decline is confined to the elderly. It's been estimated that it begins to drop after the age of ten, declining by between 2 and 3 per cent each decade, so younger people cannot ignore this factor; it's part of the whole picture. You can help by keeping as active as possible. Finally, when you are injured (or recovering from surgery), your body needs more energy to repair the damage that has been done to it, so your BMR can be affected in these circumstances too; some illnesses also have an impact. The effects are often seen as weight loss rather than weight gain, however.

If you want to work out your BMR in calories, you can follow a simple calculation called the Harris Benedict equation. Doing this will help you determine a personal calorie target rather than going for a general figure, though you can do that too if you are careful. It's a good guide, providing you are not exceptionally thin or very obese; calculating energy expenditure like this isn't a completely exact science, but it's a good place to start. You will need to know your weight in kilograms and your height in centimetres. Don't rely on your memory, guess or convert the imperial measurements that you 'know' you are, but weigh and measure yourself afresh, in metric, without shoes – and follow this:

WOMEN: BMR =
655 + (9.6 x weight in kg) + (1.8 x height in cm) – (4.7 x age in years)
MEN: BMR =
66 + (13.7 x weight in kg) + (5 x height in cm) – (6.8 x age in years).

It's not as complicated as it looks. Take a 35-year-old woman, weighing 65 kilos, who is 1.55 metres tall. That would be 655 + (9.6 x 65) + (1.8 x 155) – (4.7 x 35), or 655 plus 624, plus 279 and minus 164.5: a BMR of 1,393.5 – the calories her body needs to simply keep going, which can be rounded up to 1,400 as the difference is minimal.

But remember that, important though your BMR is, it's not the whole picture. To do anything more than perform basic functions like breathing, your body will use up more energy.

Energy out – the thermic effect of eating and digesting food

Eating, digesting and storing food also uses energy. The thermic effect of food is the increased energy above the BMR which your body requires, and it is usually estimated at an average of about 10 per cent of the calorie value of the food just eaten. Therefore, if you have enjoyed a plate of pasta and a bowl of salad totalling 600 calories, your body will use about 60 calories in processing them. It is a minor part of the whole, though, and you can ignore it when deciding the calorie levels you are going to stick to when dieting.

Energy out – the thermic effect of exercise

Exercise is a more important part of the equation, and it's also a much more variable part of the whole. 'Exercise' in this context doesn't just refer to hurling yourself around a football pitch or sweating in a gym: it means everything you do other than complete rest – from standing up in the morning to going to bed at night. Whenever you walk about, stir your coffee, pick something up, run for a bus, dance or lift weights, you use energy. Your muscles are burning more calories. It might be as little as 10 per cent of your energy output; it could – if you were a serious athlete – be as high as 50 per cent. It's not easy to say how much energy a particular activity uses, because it varies according to sex and body weight, but exercise is good for your overall health.

To work out what your total daily calorie use is at the moment you need to assess yourself. You should now have a figure for your BMR; in the case of the 35-year-old female example on page 13, it was 1,400.

- If you are a man, and are basically inactive (with a desk job and taking little or no exercise other than walking to and from your car), multiply your BMR by 1.4. Do the same if you are an equally inactive woman.
- If you get some light exercise every day – you walk to work, or part of the way there; you take stairs instead of escalators or lifts, maybe walk the dog – then multiply your BMR by 1.5, whether you are male or female.
- Now, if you take regular aerobic exercise – exercise which gets you breathing a bit faster, like brisk walking, swimming, doing aerobics – multiply your BMR by 1.78 if you're a man, and by 1.64 if you're a woman.
- Serious athletes or people with heavy jobs should multiply their BMR by 2.1 or 1.82, according to whether they are male or female.

That woman with a BMR of 1,400 who does no exercise is using about 1,960 calories every day. If she does some exercise she'll use 2,100, and that figure would rise to nearly 2,300 calories if she did regular exercise. At the most basic level, if she takes in more calories in the form of food and drink than she uses at present, she'll put weight on. If she matches her calorie intake to the calories she uses, she'll stay the same. And if she eats less, she'll lose weight. A serious word of warning now: it is very, very important not to eat too little – it can be a fine line between doing that and developing an eating disorder, which can have a permanent negative impact on your health.

Work out your own figure, being honest and realistic about your activity levels right now, so that you'll have a rough idea how many calories you are using each day. This figure is not the whole picture, though, but just one part – so try not to leap to any definite conclusions about how much you should be eating just yet. For weight loss to work it has to be gradual, and you need to ensure that your target is a sensible one.

There are other ways of calculating your energy expenditure, and the figures you get will vary slightly from method to method; there's always a subjective element, for example where you have to decide how much exercise you get or interpret expressions like 'sedentary lifestyle'. Being absolutely precise is not critical. One of the most important aspects of calorie counting is not to get completely bogged down in the detail, but to be happy with a general picture and adjust it if necessary.

Boosting your BMR

Most of the calories you take in are used to keep your body going – your BMR. Boosting it and increasing the amount used might make a real difference to your diet, so how can it be improved?

There's not a lot you can do about some aspects of your metabolic rate – you're never going to get younger or turn into a man – but you can think about the role of muscle. Remember that it uses about six times more energy than fat, even at rest, and without exercise fat usually replaces muscle. Increasing your activity will help both in building muscle, thus improving your BMR, and in just using up more energy all round. The more energy you use in exercise, the more important the thermic effect of exercise becomes in your overall energy usage, too, and that means your BMR is slightly less significant. We've seen that larger bodies need more energy just to keep them going, but your BMR will drop as you reduce in size, so it is even more important that you work to increase it and boost your energy usage generally.

Broad categories of activity are not very helpful when you are trying to push your activity level up in reality; it's far too daunting to contemplate going from inactive to active. After all, 'active' could be a championship downhill skier or international rugby player. It's much better to break it down into something more realistic and achievable. Find where you are at present in the guidelines below and try to be objective. Obviously these bands are not mutually exclusive; nobody will fit entirely into one category and everybody will spend some time doing the things in the lowest. But if you currently spend more time doing the activities in the lowest band, much less doing those in the moderate band and no time at all doing anything in the higher bands, try to shift the balance upwards.

In the higher levels you should be taking deliberate exercise, which many overweight people either hate or find deeply unappealing; it should, however, be possible to find something acceptable when you do a bit of creative thinking.

Don't force yourself to do an activity you dislike as you won't stick with it. But anything you add – particularly anything at a higher level than what you presently do – is great.

1. Low levels of exercise: resting; reading; listening to the radio, watching TV, a film or passively surfing the net; eating, chatting; having a purely desk-based job.

2. Low to light levels: light housework (dusting, cooking, washing up, making beds), driving, playing pool or darts, playing a musical instrument; typing, doing general office work.

3. Light levels: medium-energy housework (vacuuming the house, for example, or ironing energetically), pottering in the garden, gently playing cricket, strolling. Work with a light level of activity would be less sedentary than in the previous category.

4. Moderate levels: weeding the garden or mowing the lawn, cleaning windows, washing the car, decorating or doing DIY, playing golf or table tennis, gentle yoga or swimming, t'ai chi, walking at about 3 m.p.h. Someone whose work placed them in this category might be a carpenter, a mechanic or perhaps a gardener or teacher. Playing with children also counts, providing that it involves some running about and not sitting over a board game.

5. High levels: heavy work in the garden, like digging; walking or swimming briskly, dancing, jogging, doing vigorous yoga (such as Ashtanga yoga), playing volleyball or tennis, kayaking, cycling gently or doing circuit training.

6. Highest levels: cross-country walking and climbing; cycling, swimming and playing tennis energetically, playing football or rugby, weight training, running, skiing…

It is important to be realistic when looking at ways of increasing your BMR, which will inevitably fall as you lose weight. There are some supplements and foods which claim that they will 'increase your metabolism'; you should be sceptical about them. The only sure way is to do some structured exercise and increase your overall level of activity.

Is exercise really that important?

Before you give up in horror at the Level 6 activities, bear in mind the following points because motivation is critical, and exercise brings many other benefits:

- As you lose weight, you will feel more comfortable taking exercise in the first place.
- Exercise makes you feel good about yourself and, paradoxically, will help you feel less tired (people who exercise often sleep better).
- It has been shown to help lift depression; doing something physical can often lift a gloomy mood or shake you out of worrying about some specific problem.
- It reduces stress.
- It also strengthens bones. Osteoporosis, sometimes called 'brittle bone disease', is a result of low bone density, and stronger bones mean fewer fractures. Osteoporosis is often seen as exclusively applying to menopausal and elderly women, but it actually affects everyone: bone density is at its greatest in your thirties, but then declines. Three things can improve it significantly and one is weight-bearing exercise such as jogging (the others are eating healthily, with good calcium and vitamin D intake, and not smoking). Not moving about is bad for your bones, and the stronger muscles you develop when you exercise also help.
- It can help prevent arthritis from developing, and may also go some way to alleviate the pain it causes.

- Exercise particularly reduces the amount of mid-section fat, and this is the fat that has been linked to increased rates of heart disease and type 2 diabetes.
- The more muscle cells you have, the more efficiently your body metabolises food.
- Exercise can be simple and does not have to be daunting. Walking along briskly gives you many of the same benefits as throwing yourself on to the machines in a gym. Walking doesn't need special equipment, expensive membership fees or any form of tight Lycra clothing; it is usually completely safe physically and can be done anywhere convenient, any time.

It is important to remind yourself of these benefits, because the relationship between exercise and weight is complex – and you may not lose as much as you hoped after starting an exercise programme. There's a lot of truth in the phrase 'working up an appetite' and you will inevitably feel hungry after exercising, so there's always a danger that you'll eat too much as a result. Exercise is no substitute for changing your diet. Having said that, there is some evidence that those dieters who succeed in keeping their excess weight off permanently are the ones who incorporate more exercise into their daily life. People who do some exercise three times a week – and that's not hours and hours, nor does it mean heavy sessions in the gym – are more likely to lose weight in the first place and keep it off in the long term than those who do nothing when they're dieting.

You must consider one more thing. Check with your doctor if you have not taken any exercise for some time; you want to make sure you are up to it. If you have a chronic condition, have been overweight for years or have had a sudden increase in weight, also check. If you sign up to a gym, don't do anything before they run a check on your overall health; if they let you start straightaway, without any preliminary checks, find another gym. Build up gradually and never risk harming yourself.

2 Deciding how much weight to lose

Controlling your weight can make you feel better; there's no doubt that keeping it within healthy limits can reduce the risk of developing all sorts of conditions. It can also, of course, help you look better. But it is important to make sure that you are realistic as there's no point trying to achieve the impossible. First of all, establish whether you are actually overweight and, if so, how overweight you are. Women often think they are larger than they really are and men do the opposite.

There are many ways of assessing weight, and very many different charts and tables available. Sometimes these give targets that are obviously low and would need constant, punishing dieting to reach. Don't be tempted. Everybody has a natural weight range and if you manage to diet down to a weight below yours, you will find your new weight almost impossible to sustain. Sometimes these charts and tables are more reasonable, but the whole concept of a single 'ideal weight' which suits millions of different people of the same height, for example, is unrealistic. We're just too different. It's best to look at several different ways of assessing the situation, measure yourself against them and come up with a target that suits you, because no single method is going to be perfect. You do need an idea of the healthy weight range for your height, though. Once again, you have to be realistic – there's no point setting yourself up to fail.

Body fat

There are weighing scales available which tell you how much body fat you have as a percentage of your overall weight. But you don't have to buy the scales; you can just pinch your upper arm. It doesn't give you a percentage, but it does give you a guide. Pinch the flesh at the back of your upper arm using your thumb and forefinger. If they are more than about 2cm apart you're likely to be quite overweight – but you probably know this anyway. Doctors sometimes perform a more sophisticated version of this test using calipers. If you do buy body fat scales, they will probably come with user notes for that particular brand, but remember that women naturally have more body fat than men. Monitoring body fat is most useful when you are already losing weight. If your weight is staying the same, but your body fat percentage is going down, then you are building muscle instead. You can also buy body fat monitors or use online calculators, which are often designed for sportsmen and women, but be aware that there are many different interpretations of what is healthy and avoid any that don't categorise percentages by age. Here are some guideline figures for an acceptable percentage of body fat for someone who is not a professional athlete:

AGE	WOMEN	MEN
20–39	21–33%	8–20%
40–59	23–34%	11–22%
60–79	24–36%	13–25%

Waist and hip measurements

Doctors take waist measurements – and hip-to-waist ratios – very seriously. This is because they are surprisingly accurate predictors of developing serious problems related to being overweight. It's not only a matter of excess fat, but of where that fat is located. People who are often described as apple-shaped and have more fat around their middles, known as central obesity, are at greater risk than those who are fatter around their hips and thighs. Time to measure your waist and, like all the measurements in this book, do it in metric to make sure there are no assumptions involved. Centimetres it is.

It's not just a matter of assessing whether you are overweight: the risk of heart disease is much greater the larger you are, so take this measurement seriously and don't breathe in dramatically while measuring yourself. There are two levels of risk applied to waist measurements. If you're a woman, you're overweight and at risk of endangering your health if your waist measures 80cm or more, and at serious risk if it's larger than 88cm. A man's overweight and lower risk figure is 94cm, and you are putting your health in danger if your waist is 102cm or over. Asian men are particularly vulnerable, so their figures start at 90cm.

Divide your waist measurement by your hip measurement to find your waist-to-hip ratio, another way of judging risk. If you're male, and you get a figure above 1.0, then you are in the at-risk category, as are women with a waist-to-hip ratio of above 0.85. If you fit into an at-risk group, you need to lose weight for the good of your health.

The BMI

One way of looking at the health risk and at the relationship between height and weight is the BMI or Body Mass Index; it is also useful for working out how much you should weigh. Almost all ways of relating height and weight have their problems and the BMI is no exception, but it is useful and a better guide than weight alone. Once again, calculating your BMI requires a little maths, and you'll need to know your height in metres and your weight in kilograms. Doing it this way is more accurate than tracing lines on a chart, though. There are some BMI calculators available online, but it's very easy – and much quicker – to do it yourself with a pocket calculator.

You need to divide your weight in kilograms by the square of your height in metres. That gives you a figure which is your BMI:

weight ÷ (height x height) = BMI

An example helps. Get a figure for your height squared first. For example, in the case of a woman who is 1.55m tall, that would be 1.55 x 1.55 = 2.40. She weighs 68 kg, so …
68 ÷ 2.40 = 28.33

And the BMI is that last figure, 28.33. But what does that mean – and how can it help you set a target weight?

BMI figures are grouped into categories:

Less than 15	–	emaciated
15 to 18.9	–	underweight
19 to 24.9	–	average
25 to 29.9	–	overweight
More than 30	–	obese

Doctors use these bands to assess the general risk of someone developing medical problems, whether that person weighs too much or too little (both are bad for you). If your BMI is lower than 15 or higher than 30, you ought to see your doctor. There are further gradations above 30, and you must talk to your doctor before embarking on a weight-loss programme if this applies to you; if it's under 15 you are also seriously damaging your health.

If your BMI is below 18.9 and above 15, you are classed as underweight and should be eating more food to give your body the energy and nutrients it needs. If your figure is between 19 and 24.9, then you're at a healthy weight – but be aware that many authorities feel that 24.9 is too high, and that 22 would be a better figure. If your BMI is between 25 and 29.9, you are overweight.

The BMI is an average scale and doesn't differentiate by sex, nor does it allow for different builds or muscle mass. Men normally have higher BMIs than women (it's the muscle mass factor), and athletes don't have BMI scores that reflect reality. Nor, incidentally, do pregnant women. There's a different BMI chart for those who are under 18 as children's growth rates make assessing their BMI much more complicated, and there's also some variation across cultures. For example, the World Health Organisation has estimated that someone with an Asian background and a BMI of 27.5 would be at the same health risk as someone with a white Caucasian background and a BMI of 30.

You may also have a normal BMI but still be carrying too much fat around your middle, something which can happen if you are tall but have a small frame, so check waist measurements too and don't just rely on the BMI. Finally, it looks as though it is possible to have a respectable BMI but still endanger your health if you take no exercise.

Finding your target weight

Despite these considerations you can use the BMI to give you a target weight, but there are some factors you need to consider as a result of the discrepancies the BMI can throw up. You need to take your sex into account, for one, and your level of fitness – you'll know if you're muscular. A woman really should not aim for the higher end of a band and the opposite is true for men – the bottom end of a band would be too low. Bearing this in mind, decide what you want your BMI to be in an ideal world.

Now for another simple calculation. The person in the example above had a BMI of over 28. To start with, she would like to get it to 25; though she would like to get lower, she doesn't want to depress herself, knows that every little helps and has set a realistic milestone to start with. Her height squared was 2.40, so she multiplies that by her desired BMI of 25 and gets a figure – the weight in kilos she would need to be to achieve her aim:

2.40 x 25 = 60

Subtracting that figure from the weight she is at the moment – 68 kilos – tells her than she has to lose 8 kilos to get her BMI down to 25.

Big bodies, little bodies

You also need to consider your basic frame size, your build. We all tend to assume that short people have small frames and tall people have large ones, but that is far from being the case. Do consider this, because if you have a large frame, you'll never manage to turn yourself into someone with a smaller one. Even if you manage to get to a target that would be appropriate for a lightly built person, you will probably look rather odd and won't be able to stay at that weight for very long.

A quick way of judging your build is to look at your wrists. Slim wrists indicate a small frame. Briefly, if you're a woman below 1.58 metres in height, and your wrist measures less than 14cm, you've a small frame; if it's more than 15cm, you've a large one. If you're between 1.58 and 1.65m, the two measurements are 15cm and 16cm, and if you are taller than that, they are 16cm and 17cm. Men below 1.65m tall have a wrist measurement of less than 16cm if they're small-framed; 17cm or more if they have a large frame. If they are taller, the figures are 17cm and 19cm. No tape measure? Just circle the thumb and forefinger of one hand round the opposite wrist. If they overlap a lot, you have a small frame; if they meet, it's medium; if they don't touch, you're large-framed. If you have a large frame, allow for it and don't aim for the bottom of the healthy BMI weight band: small-framed people should go for the lower ends – depending on their sex, of course.

Height and weight charts

Now is the time to look at a height and weight chart. Good ones will differentiate between sexes and people with different builds; don't bother with the others as they are too general to be of much use. Again, people with lots of muscle will find that they weigh more than the chart tells them they 'should', but, used in conjunction with the BMI, it's a useful guide. If you were to do all the maths, you would find that the male weights fit into the higher part of a BMI range for someone of a specific height, and the female ones into the lower part of the range. Find your own figures on the chart opposite.

So how much should you really try and lose?

Before finally deciding exactly how much you should try to lose, run another reality check on your figures. The woman in the BMI example reckoned that she should lose 8 kilos. It seemed sensible; it wouldn't actually get her into the healthy BMI band, but it was almost there. She

STANDARD HEIGHT AND WEIGHT CHART

MEN

HEIGHT	SMALL FRAME	MEDIUM FRAME	LARGE FRAME
1.60 m	51–61 kg	54–64 kg	58–68 kg
1 63 m	53–61 kg	55–65 kg	59–70 kg
1.65 m	54–62 kg	57–66 kg	60–72 kg
1.68 m	56–64 kg	59–68 kg	62–74 kg
1.70 m	58–65 kg	60–69 kg	64–76 kg
1.73 m	60–66 kg	62–71 kg	66–78 kg
1.75 m	61–68 kg	64–72 kg	68–80 kg
1.78 m	63–69 kg	66–73 kg	70–81 kg
1.80 m	65–70 kg	68–75 kg	72–83 kg
1.83 m	67–72 kg	70–77 kg	74–85 kg
1.85 m	69–75 kg	71–80 kg	76–86 kg
1.88 m	70–76 kg	73–81 kg	78–89 kg
1.90 m	72–79 kg	75–84 kg	80–92 kg

WOMEN

HEIGHT	SMALL FRAME	MEDIUM FRAME	LARGE FRAME
1.50 m	42–51 kg	44–55 kg	48–57 kg
1.52 m	44–52 kg	46–57 kg	49–58 kg
1.55 m	45–54 kg	47–58 kg	51–59 kg
1.57 m	46–55 kg	49–60 kg	52–61 kg
1.60 m	48–56 kg	50–62 kg	54–63 kg
1.63 m	49–58 kg	51–63 kg	55–65 kg
1.65 m	50–59 kg	53–64 kg	57–66 kg
1.68 m	52–60 kg	55–66 kg	59–67 kg
1.70 m	54–62 kg	57–67 kg	61–69 kg
1.73 m	56–63 kg	58–68 kg	62–71 kg
1.75 m	58–64 kg	60–69 kg	64–73 kg
1.78 m	59–66 kg	62–71 kg	66–75 kg
1.80 m	61–68 kg	64–72 kg	68–77 kg
1.83 m	63–69 kg	65–74 kg	69–79 kg

has a large build and comes in at between 51 and 59 kilos on the height and weight chart, which she thinks is too alarmingly unachievable to be her first target; after all, she currently weighs 68kg. Even losing the 8 kilos might be over-optimistic. Many specialists recommend only trying to lose 10 per cent of your body weight at first, which would be a bit less than that at nearly 7 kilos.

A good strategy to adopt is to look at the whole process in stages. Go for the 10 per cent figure first, even if it doesn't get you into the best position on the BMI; keep that as a long-term aim instead. The 10 per cent goal should be an achievable one, and will keep you in good heart. When you've got there, pause – don't try and lose more for a few weeks, just keep your weight stable. Then go for another 10 per cent reduction (or even just 5 per cent). That would get our 68kg woman down to just over 55kg – well within the healthy band at a BMI of just under 23, and at the right point on the height and weight charts.

Remember that successful weight loss is not a quick fix, and nor should it be. The slow, methodical approach is by far the best way to lose weight and keep it off, and many experts recommend that you only try to lose half a kilo per week. Some slimming clubs applaud and reward the member who loses the most in a week, but that's not the best approach though it might seem encouraging at first. The more slowly you lose weight, the more likely you are to be making your diet part of a real lifestyle change, and one that will last. Ultimately the right weight for you is one at which you honestly feel healthy and energetic. Even small losses can have a positive impact on your health.

How many calories do I need to eat?

Now you have a sensible idea of how much weight you want to lose, it's time to look back at the energy expenditure figure you came up with earlier. Remember that calculating energy expenditure is always going to be subjective, but it's a good place to start.

A kilogram of weight is the equivalent to about 7,000–7,500 calories, and to lose the recommended 0.5 kilo per week, you would need to eat about 3,500 fewer calories than your body uses every week. Taking the example of the woman above again, and assuming she does some exercise, she would use 2,100 calories every day: 14,700 in a week. If she knocked back her calorie intake to 11,200 per week – 1,600 calories a day – she should lose weight and still have enough food to keep her fit and well. She could expect to lose her 7 kilos – the most realistic target for her, at least at first – in 14 weeks if she sticks to that ... in theory. It's always best to build in some leeway for celebrations and unforeseen events. Don't beat yourself up if you don't hit your target on schedule. The maths may be relatively straightforward but life, generally, is not.

It is vitally important that you don't starve yourself. If the figures you came up with give you a total energy expenditure of less than 1,500 calories, dropping by 500 calories would push your intake down too far. Very low-calorie-intake diets will fail; you will just make yourself ill, and may initiate a pattern of yo-yo dieting in which you ultimately put weight on instead of losing it.

There's another quick guide that helps. This one is based on how much you have to lose rather than your energy expenditure, but it does assume that you are doing some exercise – 30 minutes at least three to five times a week.

Men with 19kg or more to lose should eat 2,000 calories a day; if they have between 6.5 and 19kg to lose, their daily calories should be 1,750; and if they have less than 6.5kg to get rid of, the figure is 1,500 calories. Women who need to shift more than 19kg should aim for 1,750 calories; those with between 19kg and 6.5kg to go should stick to 1,500, and those with less than 6.5kg to lose should try 1,250 calories.

These figures should give you a gentle, gradual weight loss of between 0.5–1kg per week, but they're not as finely tuned as the more personal ones based on energy expenditure and BMR.

You may find you lose weight quickly at first. If this happens, don't assume you got the figures wrong and start eating more; it's perfectly normal and your rate of weight loss will settle down. If it does not, you may well be eating too little, so check. Then there's the other side of the coin: the weight isn't coming off as quickly as you hoped. Go over your targets, assessing their realism, and then double-check your calorie intake again – are you counting everything? Many people find they forget snacks, the leftovers they nibble or their mid-morning biscuits.

As your weight drops, you will probably find that your weight loss stalls and you have to cut your calorie intake a little to carry on losing weight. Do not panic and never, ever, go below 1,000 calories. A plateau is completely normal. One of the best things to do in these circumstances is just stop. Pause and take a break. Keep your weight stable instead of frantically trying to lose more, which will give your body a chance to adapt. See chapter 4 for more reassurance.

Some fluctuations in the rate of weight loss are completely normal; everyone will experience them. Most people have some perfectly natural variations in their weight whether they are dieting or not, so avoid weighing yourself every day. Women often find they gain – and lose – weight at certain points in their monthly cycle, so bear that in mind too. If your weight has gone down, and you've not been doing anything to help it along the way, see your doctor. Unplanned weight loss can be a sign of something going wrong.

Crash diets, dubious diets and other forms of insanity

You really want to lose weight to protect your health and not put it at further risk, but most fad, cranky or crash diets will do exactly that: just what you don't want.

If any diet promises rapid weight loss, like all the 'lose 2 stones in 2 weeks for your summer holiday' diets in the media, or makes you cut whole food groups which your body actually needs (low- or no-carb diets, such as the Atkins diet, seem to reappear every few years) or replaces meals with strange substitutes you wouldn't normally eat, then it won't do anything for your lifestyle change and long-term loss of weight. Avoid these and any other diets which are very low in fat. There are many reasons why you should do so, quite apart from the fact that you are after a permanent change and these diets don't encourage it. The heavier you are, the more stress crash and fad diets will put on your system. They are a very bad idea because of this, and there are other reasons to be wary.

The BMR is one. When you lose weight by cutting back on your intake of food, you also lose some of your muscle mass. If you lose weight fast, this proportion is higher. Muscle uses more energy and you don't want less of it or you'll find it harder to keep your weight down.

Even more destructively, your body cannot distinguish between deliberate action on your part – mad, extreme dieting – and a survival situation. You are starving, and that's it, so it will hang on to its fat reserves, slow down your metabolism and do everything it can to ensure that you survive. It's an unconscious process, and there's nothing you can do about it. This can lead to a destructive pattern: dieting, losing weight, gaining weight, more dieting, not losing so much because your body is responding to the demands you are putting on it in a protective way, followed by more dieting, losing some weight but even less, and on it goes – a phenomenon known as yo-yo dieting. You can end up much heavier than you were at the start. This happens because your BMR slows, and is the reason why some specialists say that 'dieting makes you fat'. It can do, if you approach it in this way. As you lose weight, your body will adapt, but you need to give it time to do so.

Fad diets are also very difficult to stick to; in fact, it would be almost impossible to succeed with some of them because they are so unpleasant. Failure, of course, can have its own psychological consequences – but the diet is the failure, not you. Don't allow yourself to be tempted into trying another quick-fix diet to deal with the problem. It won't work, and will only make things worse.

Some of the 'natural' tablets that allegedly help with weight loss may be dangerous; many are stimulants and can cause all sorts of hideous side effects that you really don't want. And obsessive attempts at weight loss can drift into the murky territory of eating disorders, which is really psychological rather than a problem with food.

Children

Childhood obesity has had an enormous amount of media attention in the last few years, and there is no doubt that, on average, children are fatter than they were a few years ago. It is worth noting that overweight children often become overweight adults unless the problem is addressed; in fact they seem to be even larger as adults than those whose weight problem developed later in life. They can have the same health problems as overweight adults, and start them earlier. When it comes down to it, they won't live as long as they might otherwise have done. Many reasons have been given for this changing situation. An increase in the amount of processed and junk food eaten, and in the sheer quantity of snacking, together with a decrease in the amount of exercise are three of the most frequently cited, and they doubtless have some truth in them. But what can you do about it?

The first thing you need to assess is whether your child is actually overweight. You may be fairly certain, but because children are growing, and because they tend to grow in spurts, it can sometimes look as though they are developing a problem which is then resolved without any intervention. You can't apply adult BMI calculations to children and adolescents; their formulae are much more complicated to reflect their growth, and their BMI needs to be monitored over a period of time for the same reason.

If you are worried about a young person in your family, talk to your doctor first. There are some children's charts online and figures in books, but there really are too many variables for a neat answer to your queries. Your GP may get you to record figures over a few months, unless the problem is obvious and needs to be tackled at once, or unless the situation is fine.

Helping an overweight child

There are many studies which show that putting your child on the scales or on a formal diet can be counterproductive, often leading to an undesirable obsession with what they weigh or to outright rebellion. Some children do respond, but try to avoid placing too much stress on the whole area of their weight. They may be getting teased outside the home, or even bullied, and you don't want to add to the pressure unnecessarily.

There are many ways in which you can reduce the amount children are eating without putting them on a 'diet'. Focus on healthy eating instead. Remember that children need nutrients (they are particularly important for growing bodies) and never, ever, cut out food groups, try to force a child to adopt a low-fat diet or eliminate healthy foods like dairy products. Instead reduce quantities, try to ensure that their food is as healthy as possible and reduce the amount of high-sugar or high-fat items they eat, like fizzy drinks and crisps. Another useful trick is to keep foods like these out of the house. If the large multi-pack of crisps isn't in the cupboard in the first place, they can't slip in and help themselves. Limit fast food, too. This should really be a family effort as you can't expect a child to eat healthily unless everyone else is doing it too. Most kids have a well-developed sense of right and wrong and would quickly see anything else as being unfair.

Then there's exercise. Children naturally want to be active; it's what they do. Society can sometimes discourage this, so try to redress the balance. Many studies have shown that the more television someone watches, the higher their weight is likely to be – this applies to adults, as well, by the way. Excessive time spent in front of the computer is also a factor, so it makes sense to limit screen time. It's recommended that children should spend no more than two hours a day watching television, DVDs or messing around on a computer. For the sake of fairness once again – and to improve things all round – it is best if this applies to everyone in the family, not just to one overweight child. There are other ways of using your leisure time which are much, much better for your health, particularly if the adults involved spend most of the day looking at a computer screen anyway, and children tend to imitate the adults in their life whether they realise they are doing it or not.

One final note when it comes to children, particularly adolescents. There is always the spectre of eating disorders. Try not to panic unnecessarily if you feel your child is getting fat and don't make them overly stressed about it; again, talk to your doctor. If you feel there are early signs of an eating disorder developing – skipping meals, upping exercise levels enormously, for example – then seek help immediately. This is not a problem you can solve on your own.

3 What your body needs – and what it doesn't

When you decide to try and lose weight, one of the most important things you can do is to change an unhealthy diet. If you continue eating the same foods that caused the problem, just less of them so they contain fewer calories, then you are likely to put the weight back on when you stop consciously 'dieting'. The real route to success is to count your calories while eating healthily, because we all need nutrients as well as calories. There's no point in a diet that makes you ill, but it can be very difficult to know what's exactly what when it comes to nutrition. There's too much information available rather than too little.

There are so many stories in the media – this food will change your life, that one will make you live longer, drink this to help your heart – and many of them are misleading. Common sense is often a great guide, so trust yours: the more bizarre the theory – such as 'bananas cure cancer', 'you can live on cabbage soup' – the more likely it is to be unreliable. Research from manufacturers who are trying to sell you something, whether it's a supplement, a particular fruit juice or the brand of bio-yoghurt they produce, should also be treated with scepticism. But there is also a lot of good research going on, and it's producing some interesting results.

The basics of a balanced diet

The full range of essential nutrients can be found in a well balanced diet, and that's what you need to achieve. It is particularly important when you are restricting your calorie intake – the food providing those 1,500 (or whatever) calories has got to do its job or you will become unwell. Consuming a bottle of red wine, some tortilla chips, a tub of dip and nothing else would give you that calorie total, but it would not help your overall health and would damage it if repeated too often.

Every day your body needs a variety of nutrients from the food you eat, but not all sources of nutrition are the same. You need to make sure that you get the best nutritional content you can in your daily calorie intake. Ideally the nutrients come from a range of fruit and vegetables, whole grains, pulses, lean meat and fish, some dairy products and the best kind of fats. If you concentrate on one particular type of food and eliminate others, you won't get the whole range of nutrients.

Nutrients are divided into macronutrients and micronutrients. The foundation of any diet – whether you're trying to lose weight or not – are macronutrients, which are needed in larger amounts. Carbohydrates, proteins and fats are macronutrients; they provide energy. Micronutrients, vitamins and minerals, are needed in much smaller quantities, but are no less vital; they vary with different types of food. Phytochemicals are the latest buzz – the many different chemicals found in plants. They've been known about for a long time but we are only just beginning to understand their vital role, and they are one reason for the government campaign to get everyone to eat five portions or more of fruit and vegetables every day (see page 73).

Dietary fibre is also necessary, though it isn't a nutrient as such (it's a carbohydrate, but not one that our digestive systems can use), and so is liquid. As a general rule, you'll find more nutrients in foods that haven't been subjected to a lot of processing. For example, eating whole grain bread is better than eating refined white bread.

Most food contains a mixture of nutrients, though it may have more of one kind than others. You would normally think of bread, for example, as a carbohydrate but it also contains protein and fat, a range of minerals and some vitamins. The main nutrient in a peach is carbohydrate, but it has some protein as well as a tiny amount of fat and a selection of minerals and vitamins. Salmon has a lot of protein, but good levels of fat as well as minerals and vitamins. And a pork pie has more than double the amount of fat that it has of protein, and is also high in carbs (from the pastry, which is also a source of the fat). Some foods provide 'empty calories' – they have no nutritional virtues – and that pork pie would certainly have too many calories to fit neatly into a dieting regime. There's a lot of confusion about nutrients, so let's look at what your food can do for you, and how to make the best choices for your diet and your health.

Fat

Everyone needs fat in their diet, whether they are dieting or not. It has many functions, some of which are visible – like the cushioning fat provides for the skeleton – but most of which are not. It's a source of stored energy, it keeps our bodies warm, it forms part of every cell membrane, it's a component of hormones, and some vitamins are only fat-soluble, so would not be available to the body without it … but that's not all.

Weight for weight, fat has more calories than either carbohydrates or protein – 9 calories per gram, while protein has 4 and carbs have 3.75 (alcohol, by the way, has 7). Many dieters assume they should therefore try and cut out fat as much as possible and very low-fat diets are common. But while it's true that fat contains more energy than other macronutrients, that energy is not as easily available; fat is digested more slowly than either carbohydrate or protein. It's still true, of course, that any excess energy is stored if your body does not need it and that the excess often comes from fat – another reason that has led some people to recommend those very low-fat diets. However, there is reliable evidence that the fats in your diet don't have to make you fat, and even more evidence that very low-fat diets simply do not work. Having some fat in your diet helps you feel more satisfied, gives food a lot of its taste and provides your body with a vital nutrient. Getting rid of it just isn't necessary – or, when it comes down to it, actually possible.

Unfortunately, many of us do eat too much fat – much more than our bodies need – and there's a lot of difference between fats. Some are just better for us. The bad fats, though, are often the ones that form the bulk of our fat intake, and they are the ones to cut back on.

Bad fats

The fats associated with the highest health risks are saturated fats and trans fats. Most saturated fat has an animal origin – lard, suet, meat (and poultry skin), butter and other dairy products are all high in saturates. Sausages have high saturated fat levels, as does full-cream milk; it's also found in coconut, palm and palm-kernel oils and is often used in processed food. The more saturated fat in your diet, the greater the risk of having a heart attack or stroke. It makes sense to cut back on saturates for that reason alone, and if you need more motivation remember that you'll be cutting your calories too.

Saturates aren't the worst, though; far worse are trans fats or hydrogenated fats. Fat is easier to use in food manufacturing if it is solid; trans fats are vegetable fats that have been treated to make them solid at room temperature. Many manufacturers are cutting them now because of the associated health problems, and fast-food restaurants are less likely to use trans fats than they once were, but they can still be found in foods such as biscuits and cakes. Check labels, even on apparently healthy items like cereal bars, where trans fats are more likely to be called hydrogenated or partially hydrogenated fats. Trans fats are unequivocally linked to increased rates of heart disease, so keep consumption to an absolute minimum. This will be a lot easier if you eat less processed food and fewer ready meals.

Good fats

Unsaturated fats are the healthy ones, and these are the ones you should choose; they will help your health rather than damage it, weight-loss diet or not. There are two types: monounsaturated and polyunsaturated fats.

The best sources of monounsaturated fats are olive, rapeseed, walnut and groundnut (peanut) oils, and spreads made from those oils. Vegetable oil is often actually rapeseed oil, by the way, so check the ingredient information on bottles; it's a useful substitute for olive oil in dishes where you don't want the distinctive olive oil taste. There are also high levels of monounsaturates in olives, walnuts and avocados.

Polyunsaturated fats fall into two main categories. These are known as essential fatty acids, since they have to come from food – they cannot be made in the body. Omega-3 polyunsaturates are found in abundance in oily fish such as mackerel, herring, salmon, fresh tuna and sardines, and in lower quantities in other fish. They're also present at significant levels in linseeds, sesame seeds, wheatgerm, soya beans and in the eggs of chickens that have been fed on grain, as well as in olive and rapeseed oils. Smaller quantities are found in some vegetables such as broccoli, kale and spinach. Omega-3 polyunsaturates are essential in order for the brain to function; they help regulate blood pressure, too.

The other type are omega-6 polyunsaturates, present in sunflower and corn oils, soya margarines and sunflower spreads. They keep the immune system going and are necessary for cell growth. In the past it we were advised to supplement our diet with omega-6 fatty acids because not enough were otherwise present. This is not now thought to be the case; if you have a healthy diet, you are probably getting enough omega 6. If you usually use sunflower oil, change to olive or rapeseed oil to boost your monounsaturate and omega-3 levels; there should still be sufficient omega 6 in your diet from other sources.

There's one other type of dietary fat that is worth considering briefly: cholesterol. Yes, having high cholesterol levels in the blood can cause all sorts of serious problems but, like other fats, you do need it. The cholesterol that occurs in some foods – shellfish, offal, egg yolk – has little or no impact on raising the level of cholesterol in the blood, nor can you eat 'good' (HDL) or 'bad' (LDL) cholesterol – a common misconception.

Saturated fat, however, does raise cholesterol levels overall, as do trans fats; polyunsaturates lower both HDL and LDL. Monounsaturated fats, on the other hand, lower the 'bad' LDL and boost the 'good' HDL, so it's not just your weight that can benefit from a switch. Being careful with fat will help your health, and your weight-loss programme too.

Proteins

Proteins are used to build and maintain cells, as well as to make the many chemicals and new proteins, like enzymes, that make it possible for the body to function. Protein is everywhere: in bones, in blood, in muscles, in skin, hair and nails. Proteins are made from amino acids, but not every protein contains all of the necessary ones. Some of these the body can manufacture; some – the essential ones – it needs to get from food. Complete proteins, containing all the amino acids needed, come from foods of animal origin, which can be absorbed easily and used to make other proteins. Proteins from plants, on the other hand, are 'incomplete'. To get the full range of benefits, these sources of protein need to be combined with others.

It's not generally a problem if you eat some animal products, whether that's meat or just milk and eggs, but vegans (who don't eat dairy products) need to be careful. Pulses – beans and lentils – are a great, if partial, source of protein; serving dhal with rice gives a much more complete supply of proteins, as does serving pasta with cheese or having peanut butter on wholemeal toast. Soya beans and quinoa are plant sources of complete proteins, as are the products they are used to make, such as tofu and soya milk; these are very useful for vegans and vegetarians, and worth trying even if you also eat meat. Soya products have other benefits due to the phytochemicals they contain.

Protein deficiency is rare but can sometimes occur in vegans and in extreme dieters. In the latter case it's because many of the best sources are high in fat, and some slimmers (and diets) have a tendency to cut fats more than is wise. So what are the best ways of incorporating the proteins you need into a diet?

Eggs are ideal. There's no reason to eliminate them, despite the bad publicity they have sometimes received. They contain all the essential amino acids in the correct proportions (in fact they are the standard against which other proteins are measured), and have significant quantities of micronutrients, including iron. Don't reject them because of their cholesterol content, either; eating an egg a day is perfectly acceptable for most people. Organic eggs have been shown to have higher levels of nutrients, so go for those if at all possible.

Poultry is also a great choice, but remove the skin as it is high in saturated fat, and think about buying organic again to avoid intensively reared birds kept going on antibiotics and growth promoters. When it comes to red meat, cut back on overall quantity, reduce portion sizes, use leaner cuts and remove as much fat as you can. Fish is fabulous – a great source of low-fat protein. Oily fish – cold-water species like mackerel, herring and salmon – is the best source of omega-3 monounsaturated fat, and shellfish is low in fat and calories. Fish has so many benefits that the government recommendation is that it should be eaten at least twice a week.

Dairy foods have another huge benefit, quite apart from the protein they contain. Every single one of us needs calcium and if we don't get enough our bodies draw on their reserve stock – our bones. Dairy foods are the best source; however, they are often one of the first categories of foods to be rejected by slimmers because they are high in calories. It is not a good idea to cut dairy products and may be dangerous. The best course is to choose low-fat versions wherever possible or cut down on quantities if you eat a lot; most dieters do a mixture of both. There's also some current research which seems to suggest that calcium can have an effect on your metabolism that actually helps you lose weight, but it may just make a small difference. And it doesn't have to be calcium from full-fat sources, either. Its precise role is still being debated, but don't rule dairy products out whatever the eventual result.

Nuts and seeds are another good source of proteins, albeit incomplete ones. They contain between 10 and 25 per cent protein, as well as lots of valuable vitamins and minerals. They are high in calories but you don't need many nuts to get the benefits, and they leave you feeling much more satisfied than you would be if you snacked on a chocolate bar with the same calorie value. The fat they contain is mostly mono- or polyunsaturated. Avoid salted nuts, though.

Carbohydrates

Chemically, carbohydrates are sugar compounds made by plants. The carbs which can be digested from food are broken down into simple sugars such as glucose. Insulin, a hormone which is secreted by the pancreas, then helps the glucose enter the cells of the body. The energy from glucose supplies most of the body's requirements, and it is the sole source of energy in some organs, such as the brain. Any glucose the cells don't actually need is stored, and some of that is converted into fat. Determining whether energy is stored or used is also connected to insulin levels.

Your body doesn't just need carbs for energy, though. They help to lower cholesterol levels and regulate blood pressure, support the useful bacteria in the gut which help digestion, build the non-essential amino acids which are used to create proteins, help your body absorb the calcium it needs, and aid the processing of fat ... Despite all this, however, low-carb diets crop up almost as regularly as very low-fat diets, but there's no reason to demonise carbohydrates. They are an essential part of a healthy diet and can be used to help weight-loss efforts in a positive way; indeed, they are the basis of the very successful – and healthy – GI and GL diets.

When asked to come up with a carbohydrate most people mention bread, but carbs are in present many other foods. Yes, they are in grains and in the many products made from grains, but a plain yoghurt contains much more carbohydrate than it does either protein or fat. Fruits, vegetables, beans and other pulses are all great sources, too.

Not all carbs are the same nutritionally, though. An important factor to consider when choosing grain-based carbs is whether they have been refined or left whole. The outer coating, bran, is removed from refined grains, and they also lose their germ during milling. Most nutrients are contained in these parts of the grain – 90 per cent, in fact. The bran shell is high in fibre, protein, B vitamins, magnesium and iron, while the germ contains antioxidants like vitamin E, more B vitamins and iron. The endosperm, which is what is left after these are removed, contains carbohydrate and protein, so the refined product is not nearly as good for your health as a whole-grain version – even when some nutrients are put back in, as they have to be by law in the case of white flour, for instance.

The glycaemic index and the role of insulin

Making the best carb choices is the core of all GI (glycaemic index) and GL (glycaemic load) diets. The GI categorises carbs according to how quickly the sugar they contain is released into the bloodstream. The glucose from foods that are high on the glycaemic index is released very quickly – sugar is usually the highest GI food, though on some scales it is white flour, which can bring about almost as quick a reaction.

High GI foods cause a spike in the blood-sugar level, and more insulin is secreted by the pancreas to deal with the higher amount of glucose. Basically, the higher the levels of insulin, the more carbs your body uses and the lower the amount of fat it burns; insulin doesn't only make it possible for glucose to enter the cells but also prevents the release of stored fat. Having high levels of insulin, or having raised levels for longer periods, is associated with weight gain. Diabetics need to leearn how to regulate their insulin levels, but this technique can also help dieters.

Stabilising blood sugar levels also stabilises insulin levels, and the best way of achieving this is to avoid foods that bring about a huge spike in blood sugar, while keeping your intake of food fairly evenly spaced. Eating regular healthy meals with a couple of equally healthy snacks will help to keep your blood-sugar levels steady.

Incidentally, this will help your calorie intake too: when your blood-sugar levels plummet, you feel ravenously hungry and can easily be tempted into eating things you would otherwise avoid. That's because a sharp rise in blood sugar is followed by an equally sharp drop, at which point your body desperately needs more. Everyone has felt this: eat a sugary snack for lunch and you'll be craving something else before long. The energy boost is only a short-term one, and most of us end up trying to extend it by eating something else. If you eat foods which are, by contrast, much less disruptive to blood-sugar levels you don't get this effect; your food is much more satisfying generally and keeps you going for longer.

Complex carbohydrates are digested much more slowly, releasing their energy over a longer period of time, and this means you don't feel hungry so soon after you have eaten them. These foods have a lower GI or GL (that's just another GI measure, adjusted for realistic portion sizes) rating; they are sometimes called 'slow' carbohydrates, too. The rule is simple: when it comes to GI, go for low. So how can you tell what foods have a low GI without looking them up every time?

There are some simple guidelines which are easy to follow.

- Try not to eat refined grains, like white rice or white flour, or food which has been made from them, such as pastry, cakes and white bread.
- Eat plenty of fruit and vegetables, but don't fill up on potatoes; they have a higher GI as they are starchy and quickly digested.
- If something has been pureéd, juiced, mashed, ground or processed in some way it will have a greater impact on your blood sugar than it would otherwise have. Low GI food is usually much less processed and also has less sugar and more fibre, which slows down the release of sugar.
- Whole fruits are better than fruit juice, which has a very quick impact; eating fruit with its skin on is better than eating peeled fruit.
- Straightforward rice or oats which have not been treated to make them easier to cook are better than those which have (they are sometimes called 'easy cook').
- Wholemeal bread is better than white varieties, and the same is true of wholemeal pasta and brown rice.
- The sweeter something is, the more likely it is to punch up your blood sugar.

An example of a few simple changes will illustrate how easy it can be. Drink less beer, eat fewer sweets and chocolate bars, dump the crisps, avoid lots of mashed potato, white toast and sticky puddings – and you've already slashed the GI of your diet. Now take it a bit further and abandon ready meals and sugary breakfast cereals – another drop. And so on, through more changes.

Fibre

Not all carbohydrates provide us with nutrients, but that doesn't mean we can do without them. Fibre is found in plant foods. It adds bulk to food and slows down the rate at which it is digested, helping us feel full for longer. It also acts a bit like a sponge, absorbing a lot of the water in the food we eat. So even though it isn't a nutrient, it is still absolutely vital – and it doesn't add to the calorie load.

There are two types of fibre: soluble fibre, which can be broken down in water, and insoluble fibre, which cannot. Having more soluble fibre in your diet slows down the absorption of complex carbohydrates, and great sources are whole grains like oats (particularly good), rice and barley, fruits, vegetables, seaweed, seeds and pulses. The pectin which helps jams set is a soluble fibre; it is present at high levels in apples, citrus fruits and strawberries. Insoluble fibre helps with your digestion by adding bulk and absorbing water, and is found in whole grains like brown rice and in products made from them like wholemeal bread, in the skin of fruit, the leaves of vegetables like cabbage and spinach, the roots of other vegetables – carrots and parsnips, for instance – and in seeds and pulses.

If you're not used to eating a lot of fibre, increase your intake gradually; the shock can cause protests from your digestive system, causing flatulence or even diarrhoea. It's worthwhile and it's simple: add an apple on day one, change to a healthier breakfast cereal and eat an apple on day 2; add a banana on day 4; change your toast to wholemeal on day 6 … slow and steady will do the trick. You may need to drink more water than you previously did, to help wash it through the system.

If you need any further incentive to include more fibre in your diet, then consider this … Because insoluble fibre keeps you 'regular', it reduces the risk of you developing some disorders of the bowel and colon, like diverticulitis, and you've also less chance of developing constipation and piles. Soluble fibre also seems to lower the amount of cholesterol in the blood and is linked to reduced rates of cardiovascular disease – angina, heart attacks and strokes. High-fibre diets in general help to prevent diabetes and have a real impact on rates of colon cancer. There's a lot more research going on in this area.

Minerals

Minerals are micronutrients, meaning the body only needs very small quantities of them. That does not mean that they are unimportant, however; even the microminerals or trace elements which are only necessary in minuscule amounts are vital. Minerals work together in the chemical reactions which keep our bodies going; without copper, for example, iron could not be incorporated into haemoglobin, the oxygen-carrying part of red blood cells. Mineral deficiencies can be serious and take many years to manifest themselves – as with osteoporosis, which is connected to calcium deficiency.

Eating a variety of different foods generally means that you get a good range of minerals in sufficient quantities. Food that has an animal origin usually has the correct range of minerals in the correct amounts; fruits and vegetables are a source of others and they can also be obtained from both tap and mineral water. Minerals cannot be damaged by heat or light, unlike vitamins, but they are often lost during processing. Refining grain removes a lot, and some products will have added minerals to compensate – check the packaging information on packs of breakfast cereal, for instance.

Here are some of the most significant minerals, together with a brief description of what they do, and where they are found.

- **Calcium** is needed for strong teeth and bones but is also used in blood clotting, muscle contractions and the ability of the nerves to send signals. It is found in dairy produce and also in sardines and other fish whose bones are eaten, nuts, tofu and soya beans and in green leafy vegetables. Some plant foods, like spinach and rhubarb, contain oxalates which bind to calcium and make it unavailable to the body. If you are relying on vegetables for most of your calcium, you would be better choosing kale instead of spinach, to avoid oxalates. You would also need to eat a lot more of it to get the same amount you would get from dairy products, so it is wise to take a calcium supplement if you are vegan or don't eat dairy for some other reason.
- **Magnesium** also plays a part in the formation of teeth and bones as well as in the repair and development of cells, transmission of nerve signals and contraction of muscles. It helps in the processing of fat and protein. There's a good supply of magnesium in whole grains

and wholemeal bread, beans and pulses, red meat, seeds and nuts, tofu, spinach and globe artichokes.

- **Potassium** is used to control the balance of water in the body, together with two other minerals, chloride and sodium (your body does need salt, but most of us eat far too much). It also helps in the storage of glucose and is vital for the normal functioning of many different organs, and has been linked to controlling blood pressure. Excellent sources of potassium are whole grains, red meat and dairy products as well as many fruits and vegetables, including avocados, spinach, potatoes, asparagus, tomatoes, bananas and oranges.

- **Iron** is vital for maintaining a healthy immune system and for the transport of oxygen in the blood. The iron found in animal products is more easily absorbed than that which comes from plants, but vitamin C helps the absorption of iron from plant foods. Iron deficiency is common. Make sure you get enough meat, fish, pulses, dried fruit, spinach, broad beans and egg yolks.

- **Selenium** is a trace element, needed in minute quantities. It is vital for regulating some hormones, in the functioning of the immune system and may have anti-cancer properties (it's an antioxidant – see page 48). Brazil nuts are a fantastic source – just two kernels will give you your daily requirement – but it's also present in useful quantities in wheat germ and wholemeal bread, brown rice, poultry, fish and shellfish. There's also some in mushrooms, though a lot less.

- **Zinc** is needed in very small quantities, and is another antioxidant. It's essential for breaking down macronutrients and is vital for growth. It's used in the manufacture of hormones and DNA, in the immune system, in the reproductive system, in our senses of smell and taste … Dairy products, meat and poultry, shellfish and eggs are all good sources; so are beans and pulses (notably haricot beans, soya beans and lentils) and, again, Brazil nuts.

Vitamins

Vitamins are needed in small amounts. They are necessary for normal development and growth; they help to process macronutrients, enabling the body to get the substances it needs from the foods we eat. Vitamins also aid good health in lots of different ways, preventing nutritional deficiency diseases and helping in the healing process. They occur in all living things and some of them are present in most of the types of food we eat.

We need eleven specific ones: vitamins A, D, E and K, which are fat soluble; vitamin C and the B group vitamins, thiamin or B1, riboflavin (B2), niacin (B3), B6, B12 and folate, which are all soluble in water. There are two other useful B vitamins, as well: pantothenic acid and biotin. Any fat-soluble vitamins left over can be stored in the body, while any excess of the water-soluble ones is generally excreted in the urine. You need a daily intake of those vitamins because they cannot, by and large, be stored; if you take in more of a substance like vitamin C than your body can use … well, you know where it goes.

In order to get all the vitamins you need, you must eat a balanced diet – and eating a variety of foods is key to getting the full range, because no single food contains them all. It's critical, because your diet is the only source for almost all of these vital substances. The body makes most of the vitamin K it needs (it is produced by the 'good' bacteria in the gut) and vitamin D2 comes from a few foods, but most vitamin D is formed when sunlight reaches the skin; apart from that, it's down to the food we eat.

Here are details of all the essential vitamins.

- **Vitamin A** helps your vision and promotes the growth of bones; it is also an antioxidant (see page 48) with protective properties. There are two sources: some animal products provide 'active' micronutrients which are immediately available for your body to use, whereas plant foods provide precursors, which have to be converted into vitamin A in the body. The best-known of these precursors is beta-carotene, a phytochemical and antioxidant which, for example, gives carrots their orange colour. Good sources are liver, eggs, butter and whole milk; kale, spinach, and brightly coloured vegetables like carrots and orange-fleshed sweet potatoes, and fruits like canteloupe melon, papaya and mango.

- **Vitamin B1** or **thiamin** helps convert carbs and fats into energy; it also helps to maintain the heart, as well as the digestive and nervous systems. It is present in whole grains in particular, but also in lean pork, pulses, nuts and seeds. Many breakfast cereals are fortified with thiamin.

- **Vitamin B2** or **riboflavin** makes the digestion of carbs and proteins possible. It has many other roles, including maintaining the respiratory system's mucous membranes. It comes from animal products like meat and fish, milk and eggs, as well as from some vegetables, notably asparagus, okra and dark green vegetables. It's also present in whole grains.

- **Vitamin B3** or **niacin** is essential for growth and development, like other B group vitamins – it is a component in at least 200 chemical reactions involved in the production of energy. It's been used to treat high cholesterol, but alcohol reduces the body's ability to absorb it. It's found in animal products and fish, some pulses, nuts and seeds.

- **Pantothenic acid**, sometimes called **B5**, is vital for stabilising blood-sugar levels and part of various chemical reactions in the body. You get it from meat, poultry and fish, pulses, some vegetables, mushrooms and whole grains.

- **Vitamin B6** is essential for a healthy immune system; among its other roles it helps in the manufacture of insulin, of antibodies which fight infections and chemicals which carry messages between nerve cells; it also plays a part in producing haemoglobin (the substance that transports oxygen in our blood). Great sources are fish, chicken, lamb and pork, milk, eggs, brown rice and whole grains, beans and pulses, some vegetables such as potatoes, sweet potatoes, and dark green ones like turnip tops, as well as bananas.

- **Vitamin B12** is needed in order to grow and develop normally, especially for babies and children. It's also necessary to produce red blood cells, in the processing of carbs and proteins and in manufacturing DNA. It is only found in foods with an animal origin so vegetarians may be at risk of deficiency and vegans almost certainly are – they should take a supplement. It is often added to products such as breakfast cereals, though.

- **Folate** is vital for the production of red blood cells, but is also essential for normal growth, and an adequate supply is essential for pregnant women; without it, their babies won't develop properly. Everyone else needs it, too, and deficiencies are relatively common because most people don't eat enough vegetables and fruit, and have too much processed food in their diets. Particularly good sources are green vegetables like broccoli, spinach and cabbage; beans and pulses, oranges and liver.

- **Biotin** is another B vitamin and it helps in the metabolism. It's found in useful quantities in liver, egg yolks, mackerel and sardines, nuts, beans and peanuts, and the bacteria in your gut will provide extra if your intake is limited.

- **Vitamin C** is easily destroyed during cooking or processing, but is necessary for growth, tissue maintenance, repair and healing among other functions. It's an antioxidant (see page 48) and helps to protect the immune system. It's found in fresh fruit – kiwi fruits, oranges and other citrus fruits, mango, melon, berries – as well as in vegetables. Potatoes are a useful source simply because they are often eaten in quantity, but don't peel them – a lot of goodness is in the skin.

- **Vitamin D** is mostly made by the body, using sunlight, and calcium cannot be absorbed without it. A slightly different form is found in some foods, though: egg yolks, oily fish and cod liver oil. It is also added to spreads and margarines, to some dairy products and breakfast cereals.

- **Vitamin E** is needed for a healthy reproductive system, for muscles and nerves and is fantastic for the health of your heart. It's another antioxidant – one of the best. Almonds and hazelnuts are great sources (peanuts less so), as are sunflower seeds. Whole grains, green leafy vegetables and vegetable oils are also useful.

- **Vitamin K** is used to make the proteins in blood plasma; it's vital for blood clotting. It's also needed to make tissues in the kidneys and is essential for healthy bones. Most is made in the body, but you also find significant amounts in green vegetables like spinach, broccoli, cabbage and watercress; cereals, some cheeses, fats and oils.

Antioxidants

Antioxidants have received masses of attention in the last few years. Broadly speaking, they are chemicals which occur in plants and animals, and which are also made in the body. They have a strongly protective role and neutralise free radicals, the chemical by-products of other chemical processes in the body. Free radicals aren't always damaging; everyone produces them and they are used against inflammation, to kill bacteria and maintain muscle tone. If their levels get too high, however, they can attack the body's tissues, and levels can be exacerbated by pollution or smoking. Free radicals can oxidise polyunsaturated fats in the body, which causes further damage. Antioxidants help to prevent this happening (hence their name) and are linked to a lowered incidence of cancer and heart disease. They also slow the rate of everyday wear and tear and the ageing of cells.

Some antioxidants are minerals, like zinc and selenium; others are vitamins A, C and E, and some are phytochemicals (chemicals from plants). Reservatol is a phytochemical antioxidant; it is found in grape skin, seeds and pulp, and is one of the reasons why red wine appears to have some health benefits; it is also present in peanuts. Lycopene comes from tomatoes, and is easier for the body to absorb if the tomatoes are cooked and combined with a little oil. There are other phytochemicals which have intriguing health implications, like the isoflavones in soya, or papain found in papaya, which aids digestion and relieves pain.

For all these reasons, a diet rich in antioxidants can only be good for you. Eat as wide a range of fruits and vegetables as you can and also whole grains – that's the simple trick. Antioxidants and other phytochemicals are one of the main reasons behind official attempts to encourage an increase in the quantity of fruit and vegetables eaten and research into these vital substances is still continuing.

One thing has recently emerged, unequivocally – antioxidant supplements do not operate in the human body in the same way that they do in the lab. Taking supplements does not work; you need to get antioxidants from your diet. And eating fresh fruit and vegetables brings many other benefits, of course (see individual entries in the Listings section).

Liquids

The last essential in a balanced diet is liquid. Don't forget to drink enough, whether you're calorie counting or not – but that's not an encouragement to spend the evening in the pub.

Every single cell in the body needs water: it controls body temperature, transports nutrients, is needed for all digestive functions and does much more. Hydration is vital and drinking water can even help you to slim. That's not as mad as it sounds – there's some evidence that people often confuse the signs of thirst with those of hunger, so have a drink of water before you reach for the biscuits. Then there's dehydration, which can lead to headaches, dropping energy levels, a lowered ability to concentrate – and an increased tendency to think that chocolate might help, perhaps.

It has been recommended that we all try and drink between 1.5 and 2 litres of liquid a day. The best option is water, but herb tea is also good. You want to avoid adding calories when you're dieting, especially the 'empty' calories in fizzy drinks and in flavoured waters which have added sugar syrup.

Fruit juices and smoothies can seem to be a healthy option, but they are often high in calories and comparatively low in nutrients. Fruit juice has such an immediate impact on blood-sugar levels – which you want to keep steady, of course – that it is given to diabetics suffering from a lack of insulin to give them an instant boost. They do count as one of the five-a-day fruit and vegetable servings, but only one, regardless of how many you drink. Plain water is the best choice for everyday hydration.

Both tea and coffee can contribute towards your daily liquid intake, but they contain caffeine, as do some fizzy drinks, and they are sometimes banned on GI diets. This isn't just puritanism or faddishness; caffeine can have an effect on insulin levels and hence on glucose levels too. A little doesn't make much difference for most of us, but if you are drinking a lot of coffee you should probably cut back.

Tea contains antioxidants which can be both good for your heart and may help to prevent the development of some types of cancer; great claims have been made for green and white teas in particular. The better the tea, the less likely it is to need milk – and no milk equals no calories. Black coffee is almost entirely calorie-free, too.

Alcohol

Many formal diets, particularly ones which originated in the USA, have a tendency to demand that alcohol be cut completely, at least at first. This is probably unrealistic for most of us and may be yet another reason why so many attempts at following these diets fail. Health benefits have been claimed for red wine, and indeed for other forms of alcohol (there is some evidence that those who drink a little have lower rates of heart disease than teetotallers) but too much still means too many calories and completely negates any health benefits. The energy provided by alcohol is used very easily by the body but the effect is modified if you have food at the same time, which can also prevent you drinking too much. It's another reason not to drink on an empty stomach.

Most people decide to continue drinking alcohol while calorie counting, but be careful. It's not just the calories booze contains; it also affects your willpower, and has you reaching for the salted peanuts or scoffing fast food on the way home. If you are trying to lose weight, don't drink more than 7 units of alcohol a week. One unit of alcohol is:

125ml (a standard pub glass) of wine
300ml (half a pint) of beer or lager
50ml (a pub measure) of sherry, aperitif or liqueur
25ml (a pub measure) of spirits.

You can easily reduce the amount of wine you drink by changing to a standard pub measure glass at home. If you were to stick to the current safe consumption levels, which are much higher than 7 units, it would mean that you were consuming a lot of empty calories which could wreck your diet.

If beer is your tipple, this snippet might help you cut the amount you drink: the evidence is growing that excess fat, especially belly fat (like a beer belly), is an active part of your body. The combination of protein and fatty acids which this fat generates can cause cells to proliferate, which is directly linked to the development of cancer.

If you find moderation in this area difficult, whether you like a pint, a glass of red wine, a Bacardi Breezer or a tot of whisky, it may well be best to rule alcohol out most of the time when you are calorie counting, and be very careful about reintroducing it.

Finally, all dieters have a tendency to forget the calories in their drinks, whether they are from milk added to tea or that glass of red celebrating a colleague's promotion. Don't join them!

The bad boys

By now you know that saturated fat should be cut as much as possible and your intake of refined foods like white rice should be moderated; that fewer nutrients are found in processed foods and that, as a consequence, cutting fast foods and highly processed foods will help your health as well as your diet. They don't just lack valuable nutrients, of course; they are high in what you want to avoid – those saturated fats and refined products.

There's another area you need to think about, and it's been referred to several times: 'empty' calories. Some foods have no nutritional value as such; they supply us with energy but with nothing else that our bodies can use. The most familiar of these are alcohol (ethanol, actually) and ordinary table sugar, and they have a swift effect on the system because they are digested in the stomach, immediately, instead of in the small intestine. Think how quickly you can get drunk if you haven't eaten anything for a while – the impact of sugar can be just as fast.

For dieters, empty calories are a waste and should be cut back, but don't try and rule them out completely or you may find your diet impossible to sustain. When it comes to sugar, bear in mind that many prepared foods and ready meals contain a lot, even savoury dishes – another reason to reduce your intake of ready meals. Don't add sugar to tea and coffee, and hack right back on processed foods, and you will go a long way towards lowering the overall number of empty calories you consume without thinking too hard about it. Safe dieters opt for sweetness with nutritional benefits, so try a piece of fruit or a handful of dried apricots instead of succumbing to the lure of cake. The desire for sweet food is ancient, doubtless part of human nature, and you're not going to be able to eliminate it, but do try and cut down.

'Empty' calories have more startling implications: because they have no nutritional benefits they can be the reason why some people who are overweight suffer from malnutrition. That's also true of some people who have a problem with alcohol.

Salt is another area of concern. Though salt levels won't have an impact on calorie counting, they will have a considerable one on your health if they are too high. Most salt in the average diet comes from processed food and ready meals, so read labels carefully and try to cut back on any salt you use. If you replace salty, fatty snacks with healthier ones – like fresh fruit or a handful of unsalted nuts – then you will be doing both your diet and your overall health a massive favour in many different ways.

4 How to count calories

This is where you start to put all your theoretical knowledge into practice. Remember: too much freedom and your diet will fail; too much structure, and you'll just give up because you aren't able to eat what it says you have to eat a week on Wednesday, or because you hate cabbage soup or are fed up with grapefruit. On the other hand, you will see how the freedom of calorie counting can be combined with a certain amount of structure and made to work for you. Don't worry too much about the structure because it will soon become second nature. You'll barely notice it, in fact.

Ready?

Start by going over the figures again, very briefly. You know how much you weigh, you know how much you want to lose, have checked that it's realistic and know roughly how many calories you should be consuming on a daily basis, either worked out for your rough BMR and activity levels or as a general idea based on how much you have to lose. Here's a quick summary of the latter:

WOMEN:	19kg or more to lose –	1,750 calories a day
	6.5–19kg to lose –	1,500 calories a day
	less than 6.5kg –	1,250 calories a day
MEN:	19kg or more to lose –	2,000 calories a day
	6.5–19kg to lose –	1,750 calories a day
	less than 6.5kg –	1,500 calories a day

It's always interesting to have some benchmarks, so make a 'before' note of your body measurements (bust, waist, hips, upper arms, thighs). You should also have a clear starting weight, so weigh yourself again. Do this in the morning, before getting dressed but after going to the loo. Make sure you put the scales in a place you can remember, where there is a hard surface. Whenever you weigh yourself (at the most once a week) have the scales in the same location and weigh yourself under exactly the same conditions so that you are comparing like with like. If you were wearing pyjamas on the first morning, wear pyjamas; if you were wearing nothing, wear nothing – and don't forget to take your slippers off. Scales which are used a lot or by many different people, whether it's the hearty types who go to the gym or children who jump on and off, may not be as accurate as you would wish. If yours are old or get a lot of heavy use, think about buying some new ones and keeping them to yourself.

You don't have to use your scales much during your diet if you really don't want to. Many of us have a strange reaction to weighing ourselves. We lose, so we think we can just have that bar of chocolate, those crisps, a couple of pints of beer … and this can build. If we don't lose, we can easily decide that it's just not worth it, that we are failures and there's no point. These are exaggerated reactions, but every dieter experiences an element of them. You may find it much better for you – and your diet – to judge by the fit of your clothes. It's not exact, but it might help you avoid the pitfalls of weighing yourself regularly if you think you may react badly, at least in part. Pick something that almost fits you now. A tiny bit too tight is fine, but definitely not too baggy and not too stretchy either (jeans are good, providing they don't contain lots of Lycra). Have a good look at yourself in a mirror, feel how you move in this particular garment. Then pop it to one side and try it again in a fortnight – you should notice a small difference in how it fits. Put it away again.

This is important: as you diet, resist the urge to step on the scales at every opportunity. It won't help and may well just depress you and knock your confidence whatever your attitude to weighing yourself. Everyone's weight fluctuates to some extent, remember. Whatever you do, however you judge your progress, remember that you want to achieve gradual, steady weight loss, not a sudden drop. You may well get that at first – the old story that it's mostly water has some truth in it – but it should even out.

By now, you'll have some idea about exactly how healthy your present diet is, or is not. If you suspect that you might be fooling yourself, keep an accurate note for a week of what you eat and drink, when and why (you can omit the 'when and why' for non-alcoholic drinks): do this without dieting or changing the way you normally eat. Try not to miss anything out and carry your notes with you, either on paper or on a convenient handheld device. This is a useful thing to do anyway, as the reasons why you eat something can be quite enlightening: 'felt hungry' in mid-afternoon means your lunch isn't filling you up; 'fed up' shows that you are using food to comfort yourself. If you are, you are probably aware of it, but seeing it in black and white can help you guard against it. You may also be shocked at the number of cups of coffee, all containing milk and sugar, or at the sheer quantity of nibbly bits like biscuits. This exercise helps you become accustomed to the discipline of keeping a record without omitting the things you eat on automatic pilot, like the extra-large hot chocolate you have on your way into work or the chips you 'taste' when out with the children.

Don't try and work out exactly how much food you ate or try to establish how many calories you consumed. You can do so if you want but it's not obligatory or, at this stage, easy – so don't think about that if you suspect it might put you off. For now, just use this as a guide to potential flashpoints or areas of difficulty. If you can anticipate them in advance, you'll have a head start.

Steady – the nuts and bolts

Before you actually start calorie counting you will need a few things: some scales for weighing food, a calorie guide, an A4 sheet of paper and a calculator. Slimmers' scales, which weigh small quantities accurately and are very easy to use, are a good idea. They are not as difficult to get hold of as you might think; nor are they expensive. Spoon measures are handy, too, and not just for liquids – some foods are too awkward to weigh on scales – and you might find a bar or cocktail measure useful. You will be doing everything in metric measurements. Most of us are more used to imperial measures when weighing food, and working in the comparatively unfamiliar world of grams (and millilitres for liquids) will help to prevent guesswork. Metric is also the system of measurement most commonly used in calorie guides, which you will need; some give imperial equivalents but they are far from universal and becoming less common.

Guides

There are a lot of resources available which tell you how many calories food and drink contains: various books and pamphlets, a whole raft of websites and the information on packaging. The chances are that you will end up using a mixture of sources, but you do need at least one comprehensive guide. The listings at the back of this book are a useful place to start. Above all, it must be easy to use. The easier it is to find out how many calories something contains, the more likely you are to check them before putting whatever it is in your mouth. You should also be able to locate a particular food in the categories of your chosen guide without too much searching, though you soon get used to peculiarities like lumping fruit and vegetables together or putting rice in with pasta. If there is too much time between you wanting to eat something, finding it in your guide and then discovering how many calories it has – it just gets eaten anyway. There should be as small a gap as possible between you and the information you need.

It's not a good idea to rely on websites entirely. Yes, they can be a useful source of information, but finding the right figures often takes ages and not all sites are reliable. There are often problems with unclear portion sizes, systems of measurement – 'How much does a cup of rice weigh? If I rely on the calories per cup instead, have I got a set of US measures to make sure I've got the right quantity for this number of calories?' – and just tracking down the facts in the first place. It is also important to consider whether a website is relevant to where you live, and it's not just a matter of the measures it uses. An apple is an apple but manufactured food differs widely from region to region; the figures for a chocolate bar produced in the USA may be very different to the values for a bar of the same name produced in the UK. Even if the site is a local one, you still have to check on what the calorie values mean: whether they are for 100g/100ml or a particular portion size and, if the latter, how clear that information is and whether the portion size used on the site matches the size of your portion in the real world. In practice, looking up calories online can take much longer and be much more distracting than using a booklet. There are some comprehensive sites, but the best ones tend to be subscription only.

You need to consider certain factors when choosing a book. Check what measurements are used and whether specific foods are easy to locate, and compare an entry for the same food across different sources to see how easy they are to use in reality. There may seem to be some variation, but don't let it put you off as it will probably be minor. Calorie guides are generally comparatively cheap and buying two different ones is useful; you may find that something you particularly enjoy eating is missing from one book but listed in another. They are also bedevilled with small errors (as are websites) so you can cross-check, and you will soon be able to spot these anomalies immediately. In addition, some calorie guides have other nutritional information as, of course, do some websites. This can be very useful, especially if you can find one that gives you a quick guide to GI/GL values too.

One final point: it might be easy to assess the size of an item like a medium apple, but at the beginning it is useful to weigh everything and make sure your idea of medium matches that of the calorie guide concerned. It is absolutely essential with high-calorie food like cheese, as guessing can have terrible side-effects on a weight-loss diet, so think about keeping your chosen guide close to your scales.

Starting your record

Now for the paper and calculator. You can, of course, do all this on a computer or PDA if you wish; make it as easy as possible to enter foods on your record. You also want something you can use anywhere. Make a blank table on a sheet of A4, with seven broad rows – one for each day of the week – and five vertical columns; it works best landscape rather than portrait – that is, with the long sides at top and bottom. Keep it as big as possible without generous margins; you'll need the space to write in and you can always use the back of the paper for notes. The columns at each end should be much narrower than the other three.

List the days of the week down the rows in the first column. The other three are for recording what you eat in the morning, the afternoon and the evening and will help you think about spreading your intake across the day. The last column is where you'll put your daily totals. You might also want to record your starting weight for each week somewhere obvious. Photocopy this and put the original to one side.

Go!

You've got all the information you need, but there's one other thing you must think about: planning. If you just weigh foods and write them down, the chances are that you'll have eaten all your calories by lunchtime. That would not be a good idea. Your blood-sugar levels would be all over the place, you'd be starving to death by what would have been supper time – and that would be the end of your diet. Never, ever miss meals deliberately or starve yourself; both are a shortcut to bingeing. So you need to do a little planning.

The rough food diary you kept before you actually started dieting (if you kept it, that is) will have helped you to isolate your weak spots. Your mid-afternoon snack may not be particularly associated with a blood-sugar low, for example, it may just come about because you need to get away from your desk before you bite someone and have got into the habit of popping out for something more edible. (Your mood could be the result of dropping blood sugar, though – see what happens as your diet changes.) It would make sense, therefore, to allow yourself an apple or pear at about that time (most sandwich bars sell fruit so you can still get away from your desk if you need to). This is only one example;

you're likely to have your own, so think about them and see how they can be incorporated in your diet.

Think about how you want to spread your calories throughout the day, bearing in mind that you should eat regular meals and that you might want to allow for emergency snacks. Limit yourself to two snacks a day, whenever you want to have them, and always have breakfast, lunch and dinner. Keep the calories fairly even to keep your blood-sugar levels nice and steady; don't save calories for a blow-out in the evening. If you take milk in coffee and tea, you must allocate calories for that too. If you start work early and need a morning snack even though you have had a satisfying breakfast, then your 1,500 calories might run along these lines:

BREAKFAST	300
MORNING SNACK	100
LUNCH	400
AFTERNOON SNACK	don't need one
DINNER	500
EVENING SNACK	100
MILK DURING DAY	100

The figure for milk is an estimate, though a fairly accurate one for those who take it in coffee and tea. You may not take it, but if you do you might want to consider starting to drink your coffee black and your tea with a calorie-free slice of lemon, and use those 100 calories for food instead. You may use less (or even more) than 100 calories' worth, too. Work out how much you are likely to use by measuring some milk into a separate jug or sealable container. Use that milk for all your drinks during a single day and measure how much is left last thing at night. If you have to add more, measure it first. Taking the leftover figure from the starting figure (plus any milk you added) will give you a basic idea. Work out the calories and allow for them as an average in your daily calorie total. If the figure is over 100, you definitely need to cut down; you shouldn't use lots of calories on any one thing. There may also be some days when you drink more cups, possibly at the weekend, so watch out for them. Write your milk allocation down on your sheet for each day, and remember that you can now consume 1,500 calories per day minus whatever that figure is.

You might have noticed something missing from that allocation of daily calories: alcohol. If you like a glass of wine in the evening, you have to allow for it. You can't ignore it because the calories could make a substantial difference. If you want to continue to have your glass of wine – or other alcohol – you need to know that you can stop at one, and that it won't be an enormous glass. This is where the bar measure comes in handy. Measure yourself 125ml of wine – a standard pub measure and about 85 calories, depending on the type – and pour it into the wine glass you normally use. It's not a lot. Most glasses are at least 150ml, and that's 102 calories. Are you sure you still want that glass or would you rather have milk in tea and coffee?

Two factors will make an immediate difference to your calorie intake, without you weighing or measuring a single thing. You know about them in theory, and this is where you should go for it if you haven't already. Cut down on junk food; cut down on ready meals and highly processed foods. Get rid of them if you can; they really have no place in a truly healthy diet.

Calorie-counted ready meals are tempting but do try and resist. They make your diet something unusual, not part of all-round lifestyle change; they also make it difficult to eat with your family. They aren't as good for you as the home-made equivalent (read the ingredients list on the one you fancy; if you see something you don't recognise or couldn't buy in a normal shop, put it back). Sometimes they are handy, admittedly, but don't rely on them.

Portion sizes

Another way of reducing the calories in your food without precise measurements is to look at the sheer quantity of food you eat. How big are your helpings? Think about this objectively, because cutting back portion sizes means cutting back calories. Do remember, though, that you don't want to eat too little, and that you do want to eat a balanced diet. When you are eating out, of course, never order anything extra large. Here are some realistic guidelines to aim for:

- Cheese: a piece the size of a small matchbox
- Meat or poultry: a piece the size of a pack of cards or the back of your fist (or three slices of roast meat)
- Fresh vegetables or fruit, cooked without a lot of fat and served without high-calorie sauces: as much as you want within reason, except potatoes
- Potatoes: 2 or 3 new ones; a medium-sized baked potato (not more than 200g raw weight)
- Breakfast cereal: 3 tablespoons
- Cooked rice: 2–3 tablespoons

Many diets, especially the GI diets, use the image of a plate to help you know that you've got your portions in the right relationship. Traditionally, a plate would have been mostly meat, with a lot of potatoes or rice and some vegetables. Much better is a plate that is mostly vegetables, a quarter carbs (go for low-GI ones), and a quarter protein like meat, poultry or fish. Use your common sense – it's a great weapon in your favour!

Keeping your record going

This can seem tedious and time consuming before you start, but by the time you've been calorie counting for a week it will be almost automatic: do persist. The freedom of calorie counting is great, but it's down to you to take control.

You will need to spend a little time thinking about your food beforehand, but there's no need to get obsessed about it. Here's how the person in the earlier example used their calorie allowance:

BREAKFAST	300: a small fresh orange juice, two slices of wholemeal toast and Marmite
MORNING SNACK	100: an apple and a few dried apricots

LUNCH	400: large tuna and tomato salad; yoghurt
DINNER	500: cold roast chicken with new potatoes, French beans, spoonful of chutney; fresh fruit salad
EVENING SNACK	100: a few pistachio nuts
DRINKS	No milk in drinks during the day, but a small glass of red wine with dinner.

And that's the 1,500 calories, used in a balanced way. The salad was made at home and taken to work, so no guesswork there; the other foods were all easily weighed or estimated like the apple and apricots. If you suffer from the evening munchies and would like a bit extra for your evening snack, then you could forget the apricots in the morning and add 50 calories or so to the evening snack figure. You get the idea – and there is much more advice in the next two chapters that will help, as well as in the listings.

Use the three broad columns on your record sheet to list the things you eat, with their calorie values – so you'll need to weigh and work this out from your chosen calorie guide, at least at first. With time you will be able to make some educated guesses that will be close enough to reality but for now, weigh. Don't get bogged down in detail, though. Writing down 55.7 calories for a precisely weighed apple is just plain silly; call it 55 and be done with it. Remember that calorie counting is not an exact science and that all you have to be is good enough. Put the day's total in the narrow column at the end. There you go – easy.

Really? Well, there are two more things you need to consider. One is the well-known and often-experienced phenomenon of dietary amnesia: forgetting what you've eaten and, even more often, what you had to drink. If you decide to wait to complete your sheet at the end of the day, you'll forget things, so take it with you. Use your PDA if you wish, or make a separate note (but bear in mind that you might lose it). It really is best to record your intake at the time; no one remembers every single biscuit afterwards.

The other potential problem with the record is honesty. If you eat something, put it down. If you choose not to add it to the record, the only person you're fooling is yourself. Yes, the mega pack of tortilla chips may well be embarrassing, but you ate it, so stick it down on the sheet, add up the calories (agh!) and try to work out why you binged. Check out the 'solving problems' section below for what to do next.

Finally, once you have a record of what you are actually eating, you'll get a snapshot of how balanced your new diet really is. Don't expect every day to be perfect, but look at the week as a whole – is there enough fresh fruit, enough vegetables? How's your saturated fat intake? Too much cheese and full-fat milk? Your record will give you a picture that you can use to improve your diet.

Ditching the record

After a while, you may feel that you have got the hang of this recording business, know how much you're eating, know what it is in terms of calories and think you can manage without your bit of paper. Well, give it a go. Monitor your weight carefully, though, and go back to recording if you seem to be losing too much (you're eating too little), putting weight on (that would be the tortilla chips) or stalling.

Solving problems

Everyone runs into difficulties when they're dieting; it's just life getting in the way. There are hiccups like suffering from cravings, times when your weight loss stops even though your diet has not, and then there are those circumstances you can't plan for. Let's look at problems with the process of dieting first.

At the most basic level, you may have eaten more than your daily allowance. This happens. If it wasn't over by a lot – a hundred calories or so – don't worry. Look at a weekly figure; you're probably eating slightly less than your 1,500 calories each day, so your 1,650 (say) will be allowed within the week as a whole. If you are tempted to eat less the following day, just remember that it can be difficult to resist temptation when you're hungry and that you need those calories. Again, look at the week and perhaps – only perhaps – trim a bit off each day. The most important thing is to avoid going over your limit every day. If that is happening reassess your diet and spot any weaknesses, like too much beer and not enough food or lots of white bread. Deal with those and get back on track.

Expanding your record can be useful if your diet isn't going smoothly. Add some of the information you gathered in the first, sketchy, pre-diet record. What was your mood when you ate those tortilla chips? Did you need that second breakfast because your first one was too light?

Cravings and a tendency to binge often come about when there's been too long a gap between meals. If you find you are sitting on the sofa desperately hankering after that mega bag of tortilla chips, don't try and ignore the thought completely but face up to it. You need something, fair enough: but does it have to be the tortilla chips? Are you hankering after a strong savoury taste, perhaps? An oatcake spread with Marmite might give you what you want and cost about 500 calories less than the alternative. Eat that, and then get on and do something more active … and the chances are you won't be bothered too much by the tortilla-chip craving. Once you've dealt with the immediate problem, make sure you're not skipping meals or eating too little.

Binges are a bit different. Most dieters have binged at some point to some extent, so you're not abnormal, inadequate or a failure. You can prevent a binge by recognising the danger signs; binges happen, generally, when you're bored or fed up for some reason. You could be feeling irritated, perhaps – and then you eat your way through the fridge. Distract yourself: physical exercise is a good way, as is leaving the house. You must not, absolutely not, cut right down to very low calorie levels the following day in compensation. You'll feel outrageously hungry, your resolve to stick to your (unrealistic) low figure will weaken, you'll find yourself with a craving you can't control – and then you'll binge and beat yourself up again. Stop the cycle. If the trigger does seem to be food, then look at your diet sheets. Perhaps you are feeling so hungry because you are still eating a lot of refined carbs or are chasing too low a calorie figure?

Binges aren't always about eating; they are often about other problems. Recognise what they are, deal with those you can and don't blame yourself. If you do find that bingeing is getting out of hand, diet or no diet, or if you are tempted to do something stupid like making yourself throw up following a binge, you should think about getting some external support. The line between that and developing an eating disorder is a thin one.

Boredom is a big difficulty, if you let it be. Everyone suffers from this, and it's the death knell for diets. It's one of the reasons why so many of the 'eat lots of grapefruit/coconut/papaya' diets fail, so make sure your diet is as varied as possible, packed with a huge range of tasty food.

There's another side to boredom too: many of us eat when we're bored. Don't just go to the vending machine without thinking about it and don't just pull out the biscuit barrel. Think beforehand and, again, distract yourself.

Then there are habits. We all have those, and they can have a real impact on our diets. Take the regular stop for a cappuccino between getting off the train, tube or bus and going into the office. Lots of people buy food then – but do you need to, and does it have to be that high-calorie cappuccino? It's quite hard to judge the calories in something you buy, so you may be underestimating. Walk round another way, avoiding your habitual coffee shop, and get a simple black coffee somewhere else. Do you really need the cup of tea and plate of biscuits you have after you've taken your children to school? Try your best to break the link between particular activities and eating. You should also try to break any other food habits you have, especially if they are high-calorie ones like taking four sugars in coffee or always having a bag of crisps with your lunch. It has been said that it only takes three weeks to halt a habit in its tracks – but you may find you need to cut something like sugar or salty snacks out completely in order to do this. It could well be much easier to break your habit that way.

Other dieting difficulties include weight loss suddenly stalling, putting weight on and the desire to quit. The first two were mentioned briefly in chapter 2, but let's revisit them in more depth here because they are important. Every dieter has a slight tendency to panic when things don't go to plan, but you can't plan everything and you're not a machine. Almost everyone who has successfully lost weight has had a phase when no weight came off, when they stuck at a particular level and just couldn't shift any more. Even cutting calories right down and exercising like a maniac doesn't work. These are weight-loss plateaus, and they are caused by your body trying to protect itself, conserving energy and reacting as though it is in an extreme situation; they are more common if you've dieted a lot. They also come about if you have lost too much weight too quickly and are one of the reasons why crash diets are such a bad idea. Revisit pages 28-9, and stop panicking. Eat more normally and stop going to the gym every five minutes. Don't push your body too far, but give it a chance to adapt. Some impressive studies have actually demonstrated that a break of a couple of months can do you good, so take some time out from your diet. Try not to put weight on, but don't try to lose any either.

You are sticking to your diet, but your weight is going up. What's going on? Are you fooling yourself? Well, you could be; your measuring could have slipped. Maybe you thought you could guess calorie values without weighing and measuring, and are getting it wrong. Or you could be suffering from dietary amnesia. Perhaps you set yourself too high a calorie figure from the start; perhaps you over-estimated the amount of exercise you would take.

Be very careful for a couple of weeks or so and assess the situation. If you've already lost a fair amount of weight, you may need to address the number of calories you consume. Look back at the figures on page 53. Do you fit into another weight-loss bracket now, or is your calorie figure way out? If you're sure your calorie figure was fine, consider the fact that your BMR will drop as you lose weight, so you may need to make that downwards adjustment. Or you could just be a lot fitter: muscle not only uses more energy than fat, it weighs more too, but it's better for your body to have more muscle than more fat. Check the fit of your clothes.

Reassess your target. Was it realistic? If you diet to below a realistic weight for you, you will be battling against human biology if you expect to stay at that level. There's one other thing: don't make a snap judgement. Weight varies. Remember that and check you really are putting it on over a period of time, not just over one or two weeks.

If you want to throw in the towel and give up, think before you do. We've all been there – the 'Why am I doing this to myself?' moment. Write down a long list of why you wanted to lose weight in the first place and think about the weight that's already gone – if you stop you'll put that back on and, most likely, add more. You'll feel the urge to diet again because your weight has gone back up, and there you go: yo-yo dieting. Don't waste the very real achievement of the weight you've already shed. There's something else going on here, so try and identify it. Is it boredom? Are friends and family being negative about the fact that you are changing? Actually, what you deserve is a reward for getting this far. Do something to cheer yourself up, but not anything remotely connected to food. How about a makeover? A sauna and massage? A weekend break? Make it something you have promised yourself that you would do 'one day' and do it today instead. Then, when you have perked up, go back to your diet refreshed and motivated again. You're brilliant. You have got this far, which is wonderful, and you shouldn't chuck it all away.

Tales of the unexpected

It's very awkward, but you just can't plan everything. Parties, eating out, holidays, festivals such as Christmas – they can all give you grief if you let them. So how do you cope with them instead?

The first thing is not to make them into an excuse, a reason to stop dieting. In the case of major predictable events, like your birthday or any religious festival associated with food (including Christmas), you can anticipate. Simply give yourself a few days off your diet – perhaps one for your birthday and a couple for Christmas. Don't prolong the celebrations unduly; get back on your diet as soon as you can and avoid eating birthday cake or cold Christmas pudding for days afterwards. The same applies to weddings; you could apply the eating out guidelines on page 68, but you'd have much more fun if you just gave yourself a short break. Make your diet easy for you, not impossible – but don't award yourself breakaway days too often, or there's no point. They should be saved for exceptional events.

Stop counting calories on holiday too. Trying to continue would drive both yourself and your companions insane, but do be realistic and don't go mad. Make sensible choices, avoid huge amounts of alcohol and don't let treats become normality. Get back on your diet when you get back home.

When you are eating out in a restaurant, café or bar you can make sensible choices but don't even think of trying to count calories – it would be impossible, even if you were to subject the waiter to serious interrogation. You can ask about cooking methods if they're not obvious – avoiding fried food is a good place to start. There are some common-sense guidelines below. Some of them can be equally useful on holidays, picnics, barbecues or dinner parties – anywhere you are faced with choice but haven't cooked the food yourself.

- Never arrive at a restaurant really hungry. Take the edge off your appetite with something like an apple beforehand.
- Don't have bread while you order or while you are waiting for food, and avoid white bread completely; watch your use of butter.
- Only drink alcohol when you're eating and have plenty of water; order your wine by the glass.
- Never order your pudding at the beginning, when you are at your hungriest. You will probably be much happier to do without one by the time you've eaten a starter and main course.
- Don't be afraid to ask for things that make your diet easier: sauces served on the side, boiled potatoes instead of chips, dressings served separately from salads.
- When it comes to choice remember the principles of healthy eating and steer clear of fried things generally (no chips), avoid thick sauces and anything which is obviously unsuitably high in calories like dishes which include a lot of cream, mayonnaise or pastry.
- Think before you order pudding at all. Choose fresh fruit if it's available, though some fresh fruit salads can have lots of sticky syrup. Cream is generally a no-no. The same applies to cheese which can be a very high-calorie choice, though it might be a better option than sticky toffee pudding. Water ices, sorbets and granitas are all a

better choice than ice cream, though they can be high in sugar. Having a black coffee would be best!

Following these guidelines is not so easy if somebody else is feeding you; dinner parties can be difficult. If you're a guest, and the occasion is relatively formal, you may just have to accept that choice is not a factor and content yourself with watching your intake of alcohol. You can probably avoid bread without causing a diplomatic incident, too. If there's a buffet or another element of informality – like a barbecue or picnic – it should be easier because food selection is often down to you. In these circumstances it should be possible to follow most of the eating-out guidelines. Abandon the idea of counting every calorie and don't forget to enjoy yourself!

At parties choice is limited, unlike (generally) alcohol. You can use some of the eating out guidelines to help, but adapt them. Eat before you go, but not a snack this time – have a proper meal. Only drink alcohol if you are eating something, try to limit yourself to one glass and watch that it isn't being helpfully refilled. Never position yourself close to any buffet tables, which will probably be strong on the crisps and salted peanuts. You can always say no without causing offence if you are offered food – after all, you've just eaten, so you'll be less likely to want some anyway. Finally, don't forget to dance; not only does it use calories but you can't easily eat or drink while you're dancing.

Maintaining your new weight

You are brilliant; told you. You've done it, you got to your sensible target and you got there gradually. You've changed your diet for the better, and your lifestyle has changed too. So what do you do now?

Don't suddenly assume you can eat huge quantities of whatever you want – but if you've gone the slow and gentle route this option is not likely to tempt you. In fact, if you were suddenly faced with the food you used to eat, all spread out in front of you in the style of some television programmes, you'd probably feel quite ill.

Build up your calories gradually. You don't want to carry on losing weight (eating disorder, eating disorder) but you don't want to pile it back on, either. Slow and steady is the answer here too, but don't stop thinking about calories just yet, as the time immediately after reaching a target can also be the time when everything goes wrong. Do not even begin to think about going back to some of the foods you used to enjoy but cut out because they were bad for you. The most important thing is not to go insane; reaching your target is not a licence to throw everything out of the window.

At first, add about 200 calories a day and see how it goes. Weigh yourself (but not obsessively) and keep an eye on how your body is changing. If things do begin to go adrift, get back on your diet for a few days; that should do the trick. Continue eating healthily, keep up with any exercise you've been doing and monitor your weight by either weighing yourself or checking the fit of a new, target-weight piece of clothing.

If you need a pat on the back – and why not? – remind yourself how far you've come. Get out those 'before' measurements and do some comparing; dig out the garment which was just that teeny bit tight before you started dieting and put it on. Hey – congratulate yourself!

5 Cooking, eating and shopping the low-calorie and healthy way

Cooking is one of the best things you can do when you want to lose weight. It may sound paradoxical, but it really does help. This is principally because you control the ingredients and the cooking method when you cook, and can easily make the right choices, and another advantage of cooking is hardly ever mentioned: it's fun.

It's also a way of caring for and respecting yourself and others, and you are, of course, also avoiding a lot of unhealthy processed food. You could calorie count based on ready meals if you wanted to but it would not be advisable – nutritionally, you could do better for yourself. Eating like that can be very antisocial if you're the only one doing so and it's not sustainable in the long term. So break out those saucepans! You'll also be avoiding boredom, one of the dieter's main enemies. People who need to lose weight generally love their food. You can keep things interesting if you cook using unfamiliar ingredients sometimes.

You don't have to cook one meal for you and another for the rest of the family, either. There is absolutely no reason why other people shouldn't enjoy the same meals as you do. They will probably have larger helpings, particularly of accompaniments like potatoes or rice, but a diet lower in saturated fat, for example, will benefit everybody. Healthy food is still healthy food, and it's still great for you whether the aim is weight loss or not. It also helps make your diet easier to follow; you'd need a will of iron to continue if everyone else was tucking into piles of fried food while you ate your salad.

One of the major objections sometimes raised to cooking meals rather than buying them ready prepared is that it simply takes too much time, so let's consider that in case you think it might apply to you. Firstly, it does not have to take a lot of time. Check out fantastic cookery books like Nigel Slater's *Real Fast Food* – none of his recipes takes more than 30 minutes to prepare and most can be made to work well when you're dieting as long as you keep tabs on fat and sugar and adapt where necessary.

Secondly, do a quick survey of how you actually spend your time at present, without making assumptions. The media is full of stories saying none of us has time to cook (maybe we spend our cooking time watching their programmes or reading their magazines instead!), but don't take it as a given. Work out how long you spend in front of the television or aimlessly fiddling about and give up some of it for the good of your health. There are all sorts of time-saving short cuts you can use, too, like cooking lots of soup or a large casserole and freezing the excess. Then defrost (in the microwave for speed if necessary), reheat and there you are: your own ready meals, only ones which are better for you.

Balancing your diet in the real world

We all need nutrients and we need a balanced diet to get them – particularly important when you're dieting and have fewer calories to play with. This is where you can put those basic principles into practice.

You need to bear in mind a few simple proportions, because you want to get different macronutrients in approximately the right relationship to each other. These are the current UK government guidelines:

- Carbohydrate: 47–50 per cent, minimum
- Protein: up to 15 per cent
- Fat: 30–35 per cent maximum
- You can add alcohol, if you wish, but not more than 5 per cent.

This is all very well in theory – though the World Health Organisation and some experts recommend less fat (a maximum of 30 per cent) – but how on earth do you apply something like these percentages or a diagram like a food pyramid? Many diets use the image of a plate, which is fine for one dish but not so easy for others.

Your best bet is to bear in mind the rough proportions above, remembering that fruit and vegetables contain a lot of carbs, and that most things are a mixture (eggs are protein, right? Yes, but they contain almost as much fat). Look at what you eat across the week on your record sheet and watch for repetition. Variety is what you are after. Meat for supper one day, fish on two others, vegetarian for two more, chicken for one and pasta for another, for example. If you have meat in the evening, don't have it at lunchtime; if you're having grilled salmon in the evening, don't have tuna and bean salad for lunch. If you want to finish leftovers from the day before (which would mean repeating a meal), that's absolutely fine, of course – it shouldn't affect the overall balance of your diet in the long run. Eat different things; different sources of protein, different sources of carbs, lots of different fruit and vegetables.

The UK's Stroke Association has been using a simple line: eat a rainbow. They apply it specifically to fruit and vegetables, but you can use it with everything. If your food is predominantly one colour – such as a pale yellow-beige, perhaps, which is all too common if you eat a lot of pastry and refined carbs – it's not balanced. You will soon get the hang of it. And on the subject of fruit and vegetables, they can help…

Five a day

The UK government recommends that we eat at least five portions of fruit and vegetables a day. The more fruit and vegetables you eat, the better for your health for many reasons, so do try to reach this figure or exceed it. And don't believe advertisements that promise to 'make it easy for you, because it can be difficult'. It isn't difficult, but it can seem confusing. Time to clarify a few things and throw some light on exactly what a portion means in this context.

- Fruit or vegetable juice, 100ml, counts as one portion. If you have two glasses, or a bigger glass, it does not make two portions. Similarly, if you have a smoothie later in the day, you cannot add another portion. It's one portion of fruit or vegetable drink. You don't get the same benefits from drinking orange juice or a banana smoothie as you do from eating the whole fruit.

- The same – one portion, regardless of how many separate helpings you have – applies to dried fruit. So if you have a handful of sultanas as your morning snack and some dried apricots with supper, that only makes one portion.
- It also applies to pulses. Baked beans for breakfast, one portion; salmon with lentils for supper – not a second portion. If you're balancing your diet carefully that is unlikely to happen anyway.
- And if you really are balancing your diet you probably wouldn't eat five apples in one day. That would only be one portion – it's five different things, not five helpings of the same one.
- Potatoes don't count at all and neither do plantains; they're classed as starchy carbs. Fruity jam isn't a portion and nor is tomato sauce …

So what are 'portions' in this context? Any of the following:

- Half a large fruit, like a grapefruit
- A medium-sized fruit, such as an apple, banana, pear or orange
- Two to three small fruits, depending on their size, such as plums, apricots, peaches or kiwis
- A large slice of melon, pineapple, mango or papaya – about 100g in weight
- About a cupful – also 100g – of small fruit like grapes, cherries or berries
- A small handful of dried fruit
- Three tablespoons of fruit purée
- 100ml of fruit juice
- One standard tomato or five cherry tomatoes
- A bowl of salad leaves
- 100g raw weight of peppers, onions, squashes, aubergines …
- Two to three heaped tablespoons of cooked vegetables
- Three to four tablespoons of cooked lentils or beans
- An 80g helping of a cooked vegetable dish, like ratatouille or vegetable curry

If you have a glass of fruit juice with your breakfast, a tomato with your lunch, a few dried apricots as your snack, a bowl of salad with your supper and then strawberries for pud, you've eaten your five a day. And that's quite apart from any vegetables that might have been included in your lunch – soup, perhaps? – or supper.

Cooking the low-calorie way

So, cooking is good, you have the time to do it, you are sorted on the balanced diet front: but how do you cook to help your weight-loss programme?

The most important thing, after making sensible choices, is to weigh, measure and write things down. You will soon get the hang of it and may be able to guess at some quantities, but always, always, always weigh high-calorie food like cheese, flour, fats and sugar carefully. It is easier to measure liquids like oil using measuring spoons. Ordinary spoons can vary and that variation might make a huge difference, but a standard teaspoon measure is always 5ml. Heaped spoonfuls contain much more than level ones, too, so assume recipes use level spoonfuls. They usually do, and so should you when you're assessing calories. You will also need to add anything which goes on a dish when it is finished, like Parmesan cheese on pasta or a knob of butter on new potatoes, as well as the ingredients that go into it during cooking.

Never assume that ordinary recipes and normal cookery books aren't for you (some of the recipes in diet books are just too depressing or require bizarre ingredients, anyway). You can make many of them work. When reading a recipe, check the ingredients. Which are particularly high in calories? Which can you cut out or reduce in quantity? For example, a recipe might sound delicious but contain five tablespoons of olive oil. It's obviously out as it stands; even if it does serve four, a quarter would still cost you a lot of calories. If the dish concerned really seems to need that much oil just move on, but many fattening ingredients can be cut quite ruthlessly. Take soup, the dieter's friend – it's been shown to keep you full for longer than many other types of dish, contains lots of nutrients and is easy to make. Most soup recipes say you should start by frying the ingredients first in plenty of butter or oil. Well, forget the butter anyway. Use a little olive or rapeseed oil instead. In practice, and with a good non-stick pan, you probably only need about a teaspoon, and that's 45 calories. You could eliminate it completely, and some recipes don't need it, but it does give a depth of flavour (though you could get that by using a tablespoon of wine instead). When you make your own soup you can keep the calories low in other ways, such as not including cream and never using flour to thicken. And you can usually be just as savage with sugar, though cutting it too much can affect the way cakes turn out. In these circumstances substitute fructose, which has as many calories per 100g as sugar but is much sweeter so you use less. Many other dishes, including crumbles, work just as well with much less sugar. Many dieticians feel very strongly about the evils of sweeteners, and there has been some disputed and alarming research, so you may want to avoid those completely.

Finally, when you tot up the calories, don't necessarily recoil in horror; your dish may contain 1,250 calories all told, but that's for more than one helping. If it's for four you've got just over 300 calories in a portion, and if you are only feeding yourself, freeze the rest.

There are lots of other shortcuts and tips, but most of them have one thing in common: they help you eat more healthily. They're not something you should toss aside when you get to target weight, though you might find you can apply them less stringently. Here is a selection of cooking tips that will help you to keep the calories down.

Always cook food in ways that won't add a lot of calories, so cut right down on frying and reduce the amount of oil you use. Grilling is good, as are steaming and microwaving. Deep-frying is out, of course, but stir-frying uses comparatively little oil and can be very useful. Sautéeing can also be done with a small amount of oil, and good-quality non-stick pans will make a difference to the amount you need. You can also try using an oil spray to reduce the quantity, but you shouldn't really need to – you're not eliminating all fat, remember. Make it a rule of thumb not to use more than a teaspoonful unless it's really impossible. Some foods, such as bacon, can be dry-fried.

When you buy meat, choose the leanest cuts possible and grill them. Go for back bacon rather than streaky and trim off a lot of the fat. The less you cook a steak, the more fat it retains. If you're cooking a joint of meat, put it on a rack in the roasting tin so the fat drips away; don't put potatoes in the tin and do be careful about gravy. Stir-frying is another great method for meat; choose lean meat and mix it with loads of vegetables. Mince can be quite fatty, so select the leaner options and cook it gently at first so that some of the fat can be poured away. Poultry and chicken are the least fatty types of poultry. Always remove the skin and grill or roast birds on a rack. Dark meat is fattier than white meat, but the difference is minor in an average helping.

Don't deep-fry fish, or coat it in breadcrumbs or batter. Grilling is good, as is microwaving if you're careful (it can be easy to overcook fish). Try wrapping fillets in a foil parcel with herbs and lemon juice and baking them in the oven: low in calories, quick to cook and virtually no smell. When it comes to tinned fish, choose versions in spring water if you can. If that's not possible, go for brine and rinse the fish well.

By the way, always blot fatty or oily foods like cooked bacon or anchovies on kitchen paper to remove as much oil or fat as possible.

Dairy products can be very high in calories and saturated fat so change over to skimmed milk and low-fat versions. Some are more successful than others; low-fat natural yoghurt is fine, but many low-fat cheeses may not taste so acceptable. If you find something really unpleasant, then use the full-fat version but cut back on the quantity that you eat. The stronger the cheese, the less you need, and fresh Parmesan is always more powerful than the pre-grated version. Low-fat fruit yoghurts often have added sugar, so make your own version by adding fruit to low-fat natural yoghurt. If you love the rich taste of full-cream milk in tea and coffee, change gradually, going to semi-skimmed milk first, but always use skimmed milk products in cooking – low-fat crème fraîche is a great substitute for cream. It's also relatively heat stable, so you can cook with it without it separating if you are careful.

If you want to maintain as many nutrients as possible in fruit and vegetables, don't peel them; the peel and the layer immediately below it have the highest concentration. Fresh is best, but frozen vegetables are just as good. Don't overboil vegetables as that leaches nutrients into the water; keep them crunchy and use their cooking liquid as the basis for vegetable stock. Microwaving is another good way to cook vegetables – it's particularly successful for broccoli – and so is stir-frying. Some vegetables, such as aubergines, really soak up oil in cooking, so use very little in the first place. Never eat vegetables in creamy sauces, any that have been battered and fried, or any which are sitting in a pool of melted butter.

You may be disinclined to use pulses because you suspect they will give you problems with indigestion, but you can reduce the chances of that. Rinse tinned beans (many are in brine, but rinse them even if they are in water) as well as dried ones. Soak dried beans overnight, rinse them again and cook them in fresh water. Some beans – mainly kidney beans and black turtle beans – have to be boiled at the beginning of cooking for 15 minutes. How long pulses take to cook depends on how fresh they are; lentils don't need any soaking but check them for small stones and rinse them. The more you use pulses in your diet, the less you will suffer from flatulence. They are a great addition to your meals, so don't miss out.

Flavour and savour

Fat is responsible for a lot of the flavour in our food. When you cut it, you inevitably remove some of the taste; it's why the makers of some low-fat fruit yoghurts add so much sugar. By not trying to eat a ridiculously low-fat diet, you minimise this problem – just don't add more fat in cooking and trim visible fat where you can. But there are other ways to enhance flavour too.

Firstly, the stronger the taste of the food in the first place, the less likely you are to miss the fat. Use flavourings like ginger and garlic quite freely. Lemon and lime juices can make a difference to all sorts of foods, and are very good on salads. Herbs and spices help, particularly black pepper, but don't add lots of salt. Chilli is useful and doesn't have to be overpowering. Stock cubes are often high in salt, and you may want to avoid them for that reason even if they don't add many calories; many other condiments can add to your salt load too. However, you generally don't use much of salty sauces like soy sauce, so it could be acceptable. Another strongly flavoured sauce that is used in small quantities is harissa, the North African chilli paste. A tiny bit can add a lot of oomph to casseroles and soups, and is traditional with dishes like cous-cous (the calorie-counting version of Moroccan dishes would have less couscous, omit the sausages, and have loads of chickpeas and vegetables).

You might think that cream is vital to the taste of many desserts and puddings. It may well be, but a good alternative for a surprising number of desserts is a fruit purée. Raspberry purée is particularly successful, and if you want to impress you can always call it a coulis. Blackcurrant purée packs a powerful punch, but blackcurrants almost always need some sweetening. Use a small amount of honey and check the taste; if it is going to be served with a pudding that is already sweet, you won't need much.

Favourites

You may be very attached to certain foods which you know will do your diet no good, but there's no need to make them completely taboo. It's often possible to come up with alternatives which you find just as appealing, but which do less damage. Don't forget to count their calories, though. All you need is a bit of lateral thinking. Here are some examples.

• If you love garlic bread, try the Tuscan version which uses olive oil instead of butter. Cut some slices of ciabatta bread or sourdough and toast them under the grill. Halve a clove of garlic, rub the toasted bread with the cut surfaces and drizzle on a little olive oil.
• Bottled pesto can be very high in calories as well as including some surprising ingredients (such as glucose or potato). Make your own by putting a few pine nuts in a mortar, adding a chopped clove of garlic and a little salt, then grinding them together with the pestle. Add lots of basil leaves and grind them into the pine nut mixture. Then grate a small amount of Parmesan cheese (don't forget to weigh it) and add that, followed by some olive oil – about two teaspoons should do it. It's not

zero-calorie, of course, but it's a lot lower than shop-bought versions. And you shouldn't drown your pasta in it, of course.

• Make healthy 'chips'. Cut some large unpeeled potatoes into chunky slices and boil them for about 5 minutes. Preheat the oven to 200°C, put a teaspoon of olive oil in an ovenproof dish and pop it in the oven to warm. Drain the potatoes, put them in the dish and turn them over in the oil. Return the dish to the oven and bake the chips for about 15–20 minutes, depending on how thick they are. You will need to turn them over during this time.

• Adore marinated olives? You still can; just make your own. Buy black olives in brine, rinse them well and put them in a bowl. Scatter some dried mixed Italian herbs or herbes de Provence over them, followed by a (measured) drizzle of olive oil. Cover and put it the fridge for about an hour. You could also use garlic, lemon juice and zest, fresh coriander …

There are many more simple dishes in recipe books just waiting for you to adapt and cook. Take hummus, for instance. It's so easy that you may never buy a supermarket version again, though you should use less tahini than most recipes say, and you can use some of the chickpeas' cooking liquid instead of adding lots of olive oil. You can make your own baked beans easily, using haricot beans and a home-made tomato sauce with garlic and basil … the list goes on. The more you cook, the better your diet will be.

Shopping – and understanding food labels

There is no way that anyone, however virtuous, is going to avoid branded food. It's just not possible. Using your common sense will help you pick your way through what can seem like a minefield to a dieter, but there's also plenty of information on the packaging that can help. Some information on labels is extremely useful, some is less so and some would be useful if it was only understood. But not all labels have the same things on them and sometimes they can be misleading. Also, they seem to be getting more confusing, rather than less, despite the best efforts of government agencies.

In the UK many labels contain 'guideline daily amounts' (GDA); you might also see references to recommended daily amounts (RDA) or dietary reference values (DRV). There's usually no explanation, though, so here is one.

Recommended daily amounts were drawn up in the late 1970s to specify the quantity of a particular nutrient that was needed by a certain sector of the population. They were replaced by DRVs in 1991, though RDAs continue to be used as there are RDA figures for more nutrients than there are for the now more generally seen GDA. They are benchmarks, really; sound guidelines but not exact nutritional requirements. Dietary reference values are given either as calories or as a percentage of total energy from food. The GDAs were developed by the Institute of Grocery Distribution, in conjunction with the government's DRVs, following concern that shoppers wanted clearer information. They are a basic guide to the daily levels of calories, fat, saturated fat and salt, though you may see information for many other nutrients on some products. Again, they are a general guide – and as with all such information, you should be careful. Often the reference against which the figures are quoted are the statistics for women, for instance, not men. They also assume that people are getting a certain amount of exercise.

Then there are traffic-light schemes. The UK government is trying to standardise these different-coloured flashes on the front of products, but at present almost every supermarket has their own version. Do be aware that something like salmon would get a red flash (under some schemes) for being high in fat – yes, so it is, but it's good fat so don't reject it because of that. A bit of nutritional knowledge, and you don't have to worry too much about all of this.

Never rely on the information flashed across the front of a product. Some of these claims are covered by guidelines which manufacturers should follow, but others are not. Phrases like 'healthy' effectively mean nothing and 'energy' often equals lots of calories, so always read the full information panel. Low-fat products, for example, are sometimes higher in sugar than would normally be the case to compensate for the reduced taste.

Always go by the 'per 100g' figures, at least at first. They let you compare similar products, which portion sizes or serving sizes do not. A portion of one spread might be the equivalent of two teaspoons – 10g – while the next tub might describe a portion as one teaspoon, and could therefore look as though it contained half the calories of the first one. If you buy a food regularly, check its serving or portion sizes, but remember than the manufacturer's idea of a portion may not match yours. It's fine if the figures are for one biscuit, say, but a ready meal for four may only serve two adequately. If you went by the manufacturer's serving information, you'd actually have eaten double the calories you thought you had. Conversely, spreads like Marmite have a high salt content – so do anchovies – and they would both get red on any traffic-light label. But you would be unlikely to eat a lot of either so they wouldn't do much harm.

Ingredients are listed in order according to how much the product contains. So if sugar comes first, there's more sugar in the food than anything else. This can be useful, but you need to be aware that there are many different names for different types of sugar, so watch out for corn syrup, hydrolysed starch, maltose, dextrose, glucose syrup, invert sugar, levulose … Some products contain several kinds which will all be listed separately, so watch for that too.

Calories will be found in the nutritional information panel, per 100g (or 100ml) and sometimes per serving. There will also be information about the main macronutrients – carbohydrates, protein and fat. These may be broken down; you should see saturated fat figures on most foods, for example. Most nutritional information panels include salt as well, and fibre if appropriate, and may refer to micronutrients like calcium in the case of dairy products and omega-3 levels in the case of fish.

So labels can be really helpful, and every dieter will use the calorie values on packaging at some point. It's another resource that you can use to keep your diet on track and, like everything else, checking it out will become automatic.

6 Calorie counting at a glance

Ideas for low-calorie meals can be hard to come up with, at least at first. Those calorie-counted ready meals can seem very alluring when all you can think of is a plate of baked beans or a plain omelette – again. Yes, cooking is key, but what if your imagination has dried up?

Often all you need are a few ideas to spark you off, so here are some, grouped by meals. They are followed by a few suggestions about how to put them together to get a good healthy balance across a single day. It should be possible to bring all the suggested breakfasts and lunches in at 300 calories or under, and the main courses at 400 or so. Bear in mind the low-calorie cooking information in the previous chapter, and don't forget that you can add accompaniments and snacks like fresh fruit, olives, a few nuts or an oatcake with low-fat cream cheese as long as you keep within your calorie allocation for the day. There are some suggestions for feeding children and then, finally, a bunch of tips to remind you of the basics and help you develop a real awareness of the best choices to make. You'll find more useful material in the listings.

Breakfasts

Breakfast is a must. Don't be tempted to skip it, because eating breakfast is linked to weight loss and to maintaining your new weight. A good breakfast keeps your blood-sugar levels nice and steady after the overnight drop and really does set you up for the day to come. Avoid it and your blood-sugar levels will plummet, you'll get completely desperate and be downing doughnuts by mid-morning. Keep it good on the GI front – go for low – or try protein, like an egg or low-fat yoghurt. Both options are better for you than a heaped plate of fried food or lots of sugar, but do check that any low-fat fruit yoghurts aren't high in sugar instead. Milk really ought to be skimmed and if you're still using butter, spread it thinly.

- Wholemeal toast with Marmite
- Porridge with different toppings: dried fruit, fresh berries, a few toasted nuts
- A boiled egg with a slice of wholewheat toast
- Dried fruit compôte
- Natural yoghurt with All Bran and strawberries
- Muesli with fresh fruit and semi-skimmed milk
- Half a canteloupe melon filled with berries; yoghurt on the side
- A smoothie made by blending blueberries and a banana with pomegranate juice; a separate plain yoghurt on the side
- Poached egg on rye toast
- Fruit purée stirred into Greek yoghurt
- Granola with slices of fresh fruit, served with milk
- Grilled tomatoes on wholemeal toast
- Banana smoothie made by blending a small banana with milk; add some honey to taste but not more than a teaspoonful
- Scrambled eggs with smoked salmon
- Citrus fruit salad – chunks of orange, grapefruit and satsuma with a spoonful of honey
- Home-made baked beans on toast
- Grapenuts with chopped apple and low-fat yoghurt
- Two grilled rashers of back bacon (don't use much oil when frying these; they'll cook in their juices) with a few mushrooms and a slice of toast
- Two Shredded Wheat biscuits sprinkled with some toasted sunflower seeds and served with yoghurt or milk
- Kipper fillet with lemon

Lunches

Many people find their mind going particularly blank when they have to think of a packed lunch that will prevent them from popping into the nearest sandwich bar or coffee shop. These suggestions, of course, don't have to be packed up and taken out of the house; they are just as appropriate wherever you are.

To start with, here are some potential sandwich, pitta or wrap fillings (some are better carried separately and made up when you are ready to eat them, which also makes snacking on your lunch less easy while you're at work) and do think about adding extra salad leaves. These add taste, some nutritional value and very few calories. You can also reduce the calories by eating sandwiches Scandinavian style by taking off the top slice of bread: just as tasty, fewer calories.

- Smoked salmon and cornichons
- Tomato, chives and cold chicken
- Hummus, lettuce and mild onion
- Chopped cold chicken breast mixed with chopped celery and low-fat yoghurt
- Tabbouleh – parsley, tomato, onion and some bulgar wheat; lemon dressing
- Egg mayonnaise, with very low-calorie mayo, black pepper and cress
- Chickpea, tomato and lettuce
- Prawns and black pepper

Salads and soups can also form a packed lunch – but avoid deli-counter salads, which are often very high in calories, and packaged soups aren't all good, either. Your best bet is to make and take your own.

- Tuna and bean salad (it's a dieting favourite and can be really good)
- Watercress salad with cold chicken and orange
- Brown rice salad with lots of chopped vegetables
- Broad bean and courgette salad with yoghurt dressing
- Greek salad (feta cheese, tomato, cucumber and onion)

- Celery, apple and beetroot salad
- Beansprout salad with cold chicken, spring onion and red pepper strips
- Wholemeal pasta salad with crunchy vegetables
- Pumpkin and tomato soup
- Golden vegetable soup – sweet potato, parsnip, carrot, butternut squash
- Carrot and ginger soup
- Green pea and mint soup
- Leek and thyme soup
- Chunky bean and vegetable soup
- Chickpea and spinach soup with garlic
- Watercress and orange soup
- Mushroom soup with tarragon
- Spiced lentil soup

There are more options if you don't have to eat at your desk or are able to cook:

- Rollmop herring and wholemeal toast
- Spinach omelette and tomato salad
- Warm grilled vegetable salad
- Bruschetta (two small slices of toasted sourdough bread) with puréed white beans and shallots
- Mushroom or smoked fish pâté, made with very low-calorie cream cheese; wholemeal toast
- Baked potatoes with either baked beans, grated Edam and a hard-boiled egg, or sieved cottage cheese and chives mixed with some natural yoghurt

Main courses

When it comes to the main meal of the day, you should never be in the position of having so few calories left that you can only 'afford' a piece of dry crispbread. It won't happen if you do a little planning and pacing, but you don't need to save most of your calories, either; main meals shouldn't be dominant. Leave yourself enough calories to have a pudding – yes, it is possible – if you wish. Make sensible choices, watch accompaniments and be particularly careful with potatoes, rice and pasta. Many of these dishes are delicious with a green salad, which does not have to be boring. Some pre-packed salads have interesting mixtures of leaves, but never buy those which come with fatty dressings or croûtons included (or buy them if you wish, but don't use the sachets). None of these suggested dishes should need to be served with bread, either, except possibly the mussels. And don't have fatty chips with them, though you could perhaps afford to add some of the healthier ones from the previous chapter (see page 80).

- Wholemeal pasta with pepper, tomato, onion, olive and caper sauce
- Chicken and broccoli stir-fry, scattered with a few almonds
- Grilled kebabs – chicken interspersed with onions, mushrooms and green pepper; mixed vegetables including sections of corn on the cob; lamb with red pepper and red onion – all served with a huge green salad and some raita (grated cucumber mixed with low-fat yoghurt)
- Salade Niçoise, with tuna and hard-boiled egg but no potatoes
- Mussels in wine (without cream)
- Cauliflower and chickpea curry with brown rice
- Stir-fried prawns with mangetout and ginger
- Grilled chicken breast with ratatouille
- Stuffed vegetables: courgettes, peppers, tomatoes, big flat mushrooms all stuffed with cooked rice mixed with plenty of chopped vegetables and scattered with a few pine nuts
- Lamb steaks with white beans
- Grilled plaice with new potatoes and French beans
- Aubergine and courgette bake
- Mediterranean fish stew, made with lots of tomatoes and a variety of fish
- Chicken cous-cous with broad beans and carrots

- Mackerel baked in cider
- Chilli con carne with brown rice
- Spanish omelette with green salad
- Stir-fried vegetables with tofu and sesame seeds
- Salmon with lentils
- Home-made baked beans – or Boston baked beans without the molasses; use tinned haricot beans and home-made tomato sauce.

Desserts

Many ideal puddings for calorie counters are based around fruit, which is fantastic for your health at a comparatively low cost in calories (as long as you don't add cream). A teaspoon of a liqueur such as Cointreau works well with many fresh fruit dishes instead. What you choose for dessert will depend, of course, on your available calories; some are higher than others.

- Kiwi fruit, apple and ginger salad
- Baked stuffed apples
- Apricot and honey fool, made using natural yoghurt
- Bananas baked in orange juice
- Frozen black grapes
- Low-fat Greek yoghurt with blackberries
- Grilled mixed fruit kebabs (star fruit look attractive even if they don't have much taste)
- Melon medley – slices of different types
- Chunks of fresh pineapple, sprinkled with a teaspoonful of rum or gin
- Pear mousse
- Plums cooked with cinnamon
- Exotic fruit salad: mango and papaya chunks, scattered with pomegranate seeds with the pulp from two passion fruit added
- Mixed autumn berries sprinkled with Kirsch

Puddings like the following are likely to be a little higher in calories than plainer fruit dishes, though the low-calorie principles still apply (use low-fat dairy products, cut sugar, measure everything):

- Middle Eastern fruit salad: oranges, dried apricots, prunes and a couple of dates, sprinkled with toasted pumpkin seeds and pine nuts
- Blackcurrant sorbet or granita
- Oatmeal and yoghurt cream, made by mixing toasted oatmeal, low-fat Greek yoghurt, a teaspoonful of honey and another of whisky and chilling the result for two hours
- Dried apricot compôte
- Cherries in red wine
- Yoghurt ice cream made with raspberries and honey

Mix and match

Now it's time to think about using these ideas in practice. The following menus are brief summaries, and just cover the three main meals. You can add accompaniments as you wish, providing you stay within your limit – green salad is always a good low-calorie choice (but do be careful about dressings). Use your snack allowance to help you get up to (or exceed) your five a day fruit and veg. Some of these suggested menus already have five portions, but more are always good:

Day 1
BREAKFAST: natural yoghurt with All Bran and strawberries
LUNCH: spinach omelette and tomato salad
SUPPER: stir-fried prawns with mangetout and ginger; a small amount of rice

Day 2
BREAKFAST: poached egg on toast; orange juice
LUNCH: golden vegetable soup with a small wholemeal roll
SUPPER: lamb steaks with white beans and a green salad

Day 3

BREAKFAST: porridge with dried fruit; apple juice
LUNCH: hummus, lettuce and mild onion wrap
SUPPER: grilled chicken breast with ratatouille

Day 4

BREAKFAST: dried fruit compôte
LUNCH: egg mayonnaise (use very low-calorie mayo) and cress sandwich on wholemeal bread; apple
SUPPER: Mediterranean fish stew with a couple of new potatoes and a green salad

Day 5

BREAKFAST: wholemeal toast with Marmite
LUNCH: watercress salad with cold chicken and orange
SUPPER: cauliflower and chickpea curry with brown rice; green salad

Children

A few brief notes about feeding children healthily will help here. There are some useful specific books listed on page 171 which you could consider borrowing or buying; many of the same principles apply, but there are differences between the nutritional requirements for adults and those for children, as well as for children of different ages. A great way to inspire children about cooking is to get them involved – it really is worth it, even if you end up calling in industrial cleaners.

Don't give up if children reject a food the first time you serve it but, at the same time, don't put too much pressure on them or demonise their favourite 'bad' food, whatever you may feel about it. And don't worry too much about fads. Most kids go through a faddy stage and usually come out the other side. Keep offering alternatives but don't turn it into an enormous issue. Children like interesting shapes and different colours (unless they are in an only-eating-white-things phase), so use that. Many of these ideas are equally good for adults too:

- Home-made muesli
- Fortified cereal with the lowest possible levels of sugar and salt
- Banana smoothie made with yoghurt
- A large slice of melon
- Yoghurt flavoured with fruit purée; chopped fruit stirred in
- Dips, preferably home-made hummus, with strips of raw vegetables
- A small cheese sandwich made with wholemeal bread and served with chunks of tomato
- Wraps with hummus and lettuce; roll the wraps up tightly and slice them into rounds
- Home-made baked beans
- Pasta with fresh tomato sauce
- Sweet potato and red pepper soup
- Fish fingers with peas (grill these, don't fry them)
- Macaroni cheese with green beans
- Fish pie topped with mashed sweet potato
- A small piece of chicken breast with vegetable rice
- Home-made burgers
- Falafel in pitta pockets
- Fruit crumble – cut the quantity of sugar and use oats in the crumble; more fruit than crumble, too
- A small bowl of fresh berries
- Greek yoghurt with either a spoonful of honey, a few dry-roasted nuts or some dried fruit
- Some snack ideas: peanut butter on an oatcake; rice cakes; a chunk of apple; corn on the cob; carrot sticks; a hard-boiled egg …

When it comes to drinks, you need to limit or get rid of high-calorie fizzy sodas like cola – they have been conclusively linked to obesity. Water is the best option. Watch fruit juices as well and always dilute them; milk is a much better alternative in nutritional terms. Keep children's daily intake of food as varied as you can, and don't try to impose adult worries about fat. Children are growing and need it (we all do to some extent), and small children should certainly not be eating very low-fat dairy products or drinking skimmed milk.

Tips, new ideas and reminders

Set yourself up for success and make things easy. The more straightforward you can make your diet, the more likely you are to succeed – but the more flexible it is, the more likely it is to work, too. Remember: lifestyle change and not quick fix.

People who have lost weight and kept it off have many shortcuts – things that they bring to mind almost unconsciously. As you progress you will become more and more calorie-aware and be able to make the right, nutritionally sound, decisions at a glance. In the meantime, here's some help. Go back for more detail on some of these; some are new ideas and some are simple snippets. There's more on low-calorie cooking in chapter 5 and quick calorie guides for many specific foods can be found in the listings. Off we go …

Food and drink for your diet

Get rid of rubbish. Many things we eat don't supply us with enough nutrients in return for the calories they contain, so ditch them.

High in fat generally equals high in calories: cheese, full-cream milk, cream, pork crackling, chicken skin, crisps, butter on a scone – all worth cutting, and for many reasons as well as weight loss. Change to skimmed milk and low-fat dairy products (but watch for sneaky sugars in some, like fruit yoghurt and yoghurt drinks). The more fat in meat, the more calories it contains.

Reduce your intake of red meat and eat fish more often. White fish has fewer calories than oily fish but it also has lower levels of beneficial omega-3 fatty acids. Don't rule out fish like salmon because they have more calories; just cook them carefully.

High in sugar often equals high in calories but ready-to-eat dried apricots, for instance, contain more sugar weight for weight than carrot cake. However, 100g of dried apricots would be quite a lot; 100g of carrot cake would be a small slice, if that. Plus there are more nutritional benefits in the apricots (and some nutritional negatives in the cake, especially if it's not home-made), and they are lower GI too. They won't have the same negative impact on your system… and that matters, because you need to keep your blood sugar and insulin levels steady to give you the best shot at success.

Go for low – the lower the GI, the better for you and your diet. Think wholegrains, fruits, vegetables; replace white bread with wholemeal , white pasta with wholemeal and white rice with brown.

Cut out any sugar you add to either food or drinks. Change gradually if you find it hard, but completely removing sugar is often more effective than being gentle with yourself and doing it gradually. If you habitually add a lot of sugar to fruit then cut that too; you will find that fruits such as strawberries taste much sweeter if you take them out of the fridge and let them warm up before you eat them. Cakes, pastries (whether they are savoury or sweet), sweets – all worth cutting. It will be easier to lose weight without them.

Anything that boasts that it 'gives you energy' does exactly what it says on the label – calories are a measure of energy, remember. What it's giving you are calories, sometimes lots of them. Beware the sports drink; it's designed to deliver glucose swiftly to the bloodstream.

Reducing portion sizes means a reduction in calories, but don't cut them too much. It's always better to have a large helping of something which is low in calories and healthy, than a small helping of high-calorie unhealthy food.

Adjusting proportions within dishes can help your diet. When preparing a dish like stuffed vegetables, make sure that the stuffing is more vegetable than rice. Always use more of low-calorie ingredients, less of high-calorie ones and bulk out potentially high-calorie choices like muesli with low-cal fillers such as chopped apple.

Monitoring yourself

Slow and sure wins the race, so don't push yourself too far. And don't weigh yourself more than once a week. Keep a record of your weight if you want to, and if you are certain that any wobbles won't discourage you. Just aim for a gradual reduction. Think about how you will incorporate difficult situations or any potential diet-busting events into your life in advance wherever possible. You can anticipate days you have to spend travelling and if you know you have a leaving party or a child's birthday celebration coming up, you can plan for that too. You might cut back a little bit the day before, perhaps, and a little the day afterwards – but never leave yourself hungry. There are many things you can do if you just bear in mind the general principles. Check the 'eating out' guidelines on pages 67–9: they can be applied to many events.

If you crack and give into cravings or binges, forgive yourself. Over-indulging can be a sign that something's gone a bit adrift; you may have been eating too little or not the right food to keep you satisfied. Review the situation, make adjustments and never, ever starve yourself the following day. Never, ever starve yourself at all.

If you know you have the willpower of a maggot in some situations, don't court disaster. Make it as easy as possible. Keep high-calorie temptations out of your kitchen if you can't resist them, for instance, and don't keep sweets in the car.

Try not to indulge in comfort or stress eating. Chocolate, alas, will not solve problems – so do try and work out what's at the bottom of these situations that you find tend to be a problem.

Keeping the record

Don't nitpick when calorie counting, writing down tiny fractions. There's no need to, you don't have to be that obsessive about it. But don't forget to write things down either; ensure dietary amnesia doesn't affect you.

Make sure any snacks fit into your daily calorie allowance, and be particularly careful about their quality. It's not just crisps and savoury snacks; many others, like biscuits, can be high in things you don't want – including calories. If you weaken at work, make sure you have a piece of fruit to hand or alternatively you could carry some dried fruit in a small container.

In case you need any more motivation to be careful at parties, think about the calories in some party foods: mini tartlets, 70–90 calories each; mini scotch eggs, about 70; mini pork pies are a horrendous

175–200 calories; little sausage rolls, about 130 calories each; one baby vol-au-vent, up to 125 calories. A couple of handfuls of crisps would be about 25g – 130 calories or so. Olives (3 calories each) are a particularly successful alternative to peanuts (300 calories for a large handful). Small Indian snacks – mini samosas, little onion bhajis – are sometimes even worse. Even the (apparently) innocent little canapés are scary (the bread on which they are based is frequently fried). And that's before you even think about adding alcohol.

Cooking and eating

If you don't like something, you don't have to eat it: that's the advantage of calorie counting. There's also a downside, though. If you only like beer and crisps, you could – in theory – lose some weight by drinking fewer pints and eating fewer packets of salt and vinegar. You would make yourself ill in the process, and any weight you lost would return. Dieting healthily, changing your lifestyle, should keep your lost weight from coming back.

One tip which some people find useful is to eat more slowly. Take your time and enjoy your food; you will find it more satisfying than you would if you raced at your meals. And stop eating when you are full; you don't have to eat everything on your plate, whatever your mother said. One reason why eating more slowly works is that it's easier to recognise the point at which you have actually had enough when you're paying attention.

Never order anything in large, jumbo, supersize, mega – whatever it's called, avoid it.

Mayonnaise can be nightmarishly high in calories and saturated fat. Always use a low-calorie one or find a substitute, and don't use it as an alternative to butter in sandwich fillings. Avoid other rich salad dressings; the calories can be put to better use.

Soup is fantastic for dieters, and is easy to keep low in calories. It really does fill you up, and is also very easy to make. Add extra salad to your sandwiches or wraps, too, and extra vegetables to soups and stews. Pulses can also be a useful addition.

Shopping

Be canny. Food manufacturers want us to buy their products, whatever they are. In many cases they will exploit weaknesses, sow doubt and confusion and do whatever they have to do in order to maintain and increase their market share. New products, new ways of marketing, new ways of retailing and display all have one aim: to make us buy. Manufacturers do not create a highly processed convenience food which will 'save you time' because they care about you; they're doing it to make money. So try not to fall into any traps. And never shop for food on an empty stomach. It's not a myth, it really can make a difference.

As a general rule of thumb when checking labels, make sure you read the ingredients or the nutritional information rather than going by anything flashed across the front. Make sure you compare 'per 100g' figures from brand to brand rather than going by portion sizes, which may not match.

You can tell if something is highly processed (and should be avoided) by reading the ingredients if you're not sure. There's a saying: if you can't pick it, dig it or kill it, don't eat it. So if there are great lists of substances with long chemical names, it's not a good sign. Another rule of thumb: the longer the list, the more processed the food – but bear in mind that some goods, like breakfast cereals, are fortified with additional vitamins and minerals. If the ingredients list says something along the lines of 'durum wheat semolina, pasteurised egg' then you're by and large all right. That's egg pasta, by the way, so you would still need to be careful about quantities.

One final note

Dieting can often change more than your weight for the better, and when you go for the sensible, slow and steady approach you have time to adapt. So what sort of changes have successful dieters reported? Well, not only do people feel fitter and healthier, they also feel better about themselves all round; they are much more comfortable in their skin. They are often much more confident, too. Have fun!

Listings

In these listings you will find calorie values for many different basic types of food and drink, together with some information about any particularly useful, interesting or unusual nutrients they contain. Basically, vegetables, fruits, grains – and the products made from them – have the highest levels of complex carbohydrates, while meat, fish and dairy products have the highest levels of protein; macronutrients like these are not always mentioned in the listings. More information can be found in Chapter 3.

Most of the figures here are for uncooked weights of the food concerned, unless otherwise stated.

Ackee

172 cals/100g.

Ackee is a tropical fruit, and outside the West Indies it is usually available canned rather than fresh. It is rich in vitamin C.

Alcohol

see BEERS, CIDER, LIQUEURS, PORT, SHERRY, SPIRITS, VERMOUTH, WINE

Almonds

630 calories for 100g of whole kernels; about 13 per nut. Ground almonds have about 615 calories to 100g.

Almonds are a useful source of the B vitamins and vitamin E, as well as numerous minerals. They're also a hugely rich source of calcium.

Anchovies

A small tin is 50g – 96 calories when drained.

The calcium content of anchovies is good because you eat their fine bones, and they contain plenty of vitamin B12 as well. They are high in salt, but since only a few are eaten at one time the benefits outweigh the risks. Blot drained anchovies with kitchen paper to soak up as much of the oil as possible.

Apples

A medium apple is 50–55 calories and a 200g cooking apple, with skin, is 70 calories. Dried apple rings are 238 cals/100g.

Apples have a low GI, are high in fibre (especially if you eat the skin) and contain quercetin. This antioxidant phytochemical has been linked to lowering blood cholesterol and is thought to have other significant health benefits. Apples can be a good source of vitamin C, but the level they contain depends on how long they have been stored.

Apricots

A fresh apricot has 16 calories and an average dried one has 10.

Apricots also have a low GI and are high in the antioxidant beta-carotene. The dried ones are a particularly good source of fibre, but try to find unsulphurated ones (they have a darker colour) as they're better for you, especially if you have asthma or allergies.

Artichoke, globe
A globe artichoke has 18 calories.
Artichokes are a useful source of folate and potassium and contain cynarin, which seems to help liver function.

Artichoke, Jerusalem
77 cals/100g; boiled, 41.
Some people find that they suffer from wind after eating Jerusalem artichokes, but it's not universal – try them and see; they contain useful levels of potassium.

Asparagus
25 cals/100g – about 6 or 7 spears.
Be careful what you serve asparagus with: avoid lots of butter or high-calorie sauces. Nutritionally it's a very good source of beta-carotene, folate (100g provides 75 per cent of the RDA), vitamins C and E, and potassium. It contains a kind of fibre that helps healthy bowel function and is also a natural diuretic that can relieve fluid retention.

Aubergine
A medium aubergine is 300g and they have only 15 calories per 100g.
Aubergines soak up fat in cooking, so be aware of this and monitor how much you use. They have a range of vitamins and minerals, but not at high levels.

Avocado
190 cals/100g. Half a medium to large avocado is 160 calories.
Avocados contain a lot of monounsaturated fats – the 'right' fats – and are an excellent source of vitamin E. They also have significant amounts of vitamin B6 and potassium, as well as other vitamins and minerals.

Bacon

Two thick rashers of back bacon are 100g raw weight: 215 calories. Dry-fry them (cook in a frying pan with no extra fat) and their weight drops to 35g, and dry-fried bacon is 295 calories per 100g – so that's 103 calories. Streaky bacon is 276 cals/100g, raw.

Like most meat, bacon is a great source of zinc and B vitamins. It can be very high in fat and calories, however, depending on how it is cooked – dry-frying and grilling are the best options. The fat is slightly higher in monounsaturates than saturates, but you should still remove a lot of it before cooking to cut the calories. Bacon is high in salt because it is cured, so consider this if you have high blood pressure.

Bagels

About 190 calories for a plain, fresh bagel (70g).

Some brands can be higher than this, so check the packaging and eat bagels in moderation. Watch fillings, too. The traditional smoked salmon and cream cheese filling is not a good idea, for example; it would be better to substitute dill pickle for the cheese.

Bamboo shoots

Canned, 12 cals/100g.

These are a useful source of vitamin C and also contain some minerals.

Bananas

A medium one has 100 calories.

Bananas are great for dieters, partly because they are just so convenient. They rarely cause allergic reactions and are easily carried. They are also high in potassium and a source of vitamin B6.

Beans

There are many different beans. Here are the calorie values per 100g for some of the most popular ones: Aduki beans, dried: 304 calories. Blackeye, dried: 311. Borlotti, canned and drained: 103. Butter beans, dried, 312; canned and drained, 77. Cannellini, canned and drained: 84. Flageolet, canned and drained: 72. Haricot, dried, 324; canned and drained: 69. Mung, dried, 279. Red kidney beans, dried, 266; canned and drained, 100. A small tin (150g) of baked beans has 105 calories.

Pulses have been described as 'the perfect food'. They are high in fibre, especially soluble fibre, high in proteins and complex carbs (they therefore have a low GI) but low in fat. In addition, they contain significant amounts of B vitamins, folate, iron, beta-carotene and calcium. Beans are often canned in brine and can be salty, so drain and rinse them well. With dried beans, follow the soaking and cooking instructions and always cook them in fresh water, then flatulence shouldn't be a problem. Baked beans in tomato sauce also contain the antioxidant lycopene from the tomatoes, but can be high in sugar and salt – check the nutritional information on the can.

see also LENTILS AND CHICKPEAS, GREEN OR FRENCH BEANS, RUNNER BEANS

Beansprouts

31 cals/100g.

Beansprouts are a great source of vitamin C and contain useful quantities of B vitamins (thiamin, folate and B6). They also provide protein in an easily digested form.

Beef

Lean beef has 152 calories to 100g raw weight, and minced beef is 252 calories/100g. Stewing steak, lean and fat, has 164. A small fillet steak is about 225g raw weight – 310 calories. A rump steak the same size has 286 and a sirloin steak has 325. How steak is cooked affects calorie content: well-cooked steaks are lower than rare ones. And, as a general guide, a burger which is 50g raw weight has 145 calories.

Beef is a good source of B vitamins, iron and zinc and other minerals, but the quantity is variable and often depends on how the animal was raised. Cooking methods are important – trim fat, cook joints on a rack rather than sitting them in a roasting tin, grill cuts like steaks. Commercial beef products like burgers are often high in fat, preservatives and other additives, so go for the best quality you can afford, cook them well and don't add extra fat.

....

Beers

As an average, expect half a pint of beer to contain 92 calories and a pint (of course) double that. Lager is 83 for a half; Guinness, 83; premium lagers on average are 162 per bottle. Barley wine is 181.

Dark beers and stouts contain more phytochemicals than light ones, as well as some minerals and vitamins. They also contain a lot of calories, as do all beers, so watch your consumption carefully.

....

Beetroot

36 cals/100g. Pickled beetroot, 28 cals/100g.

Beetroot is a great source of folate, is high in potassium and contains some vitamin C. Try roasting it – delicious. It is also tasty in a home-made vegetable juice, combined with carrot and celery, or in the Eastern European soup borscht.

see also SWISS CHARD AND LEAF BEET

....

Biscuits

Biscuits vary enormously, so check packaging – a chocolate chip cookie can be 115 calories; a Morning Coffee biscuit, 25. An average chocolate digestive is 89, a plain one 71, and a Ginger Nut 46. Flapjacks have 493 cals to 100g on average.

Many biscuits are high in sugar and saturated fat and sometimes in trans fats. Salt levels can also be surprisingly high, even in sweet biscuits – check out digestives, for instance. They're all generally low in fibre, vitamins and minerals.

....

Blackberries

25 cals/100g – a bowlful.

Blackberries are a useful source of vitamin C, folate and vitamin E. They also contain valuable bioflavonoids, which seem to block the action of cancer cells. If you pick them rather than buy them, make sure it's not from a potentially polluted site as their soft skins will absorb pollutants.

Blackcurrants and redcurrants

Blackcurrants are 28 cals/100g; redcurrants, 24.

Blackcurrants, raw, contain four times as much vitamin C as an orange – about 200mg per 100g. Cooking reduces this level, but they're still high. They also contain anthocyanins, which give them their colour and which are valuable antioxidants. Redcurrants aren't as high in vitamin C, but still contain more than most fruit. Both are good sources of fibre and iron.

Blueberries and bilberries

Fresh, they have about 30 cals/100g; dried blueberries, 330.

These can be eaten raw, preserving their vitamin C. Like blackcurrants, they contain fibre, iron and anthocyanins, which have many health benefits and have led to blueberries being dubbed a 'superfood'.

Brazil nuts

682 cals/100g – about 25 per nut.

Brazil nuts are high in fat, but they are also spectacularly good sources of selenium, which works as an antioxidant. They are high in vitamins B and E, magnesium, iodine and phosphorus. The fat they contain is mostly mono- or polyunsaturated.

Bread

Slices vary in size and thickness, so these figures are for 100g. Check weights until you get used to the size of slice you generally use; a medium one is usually about 35g. Brown bread, 207; granary, 237; rye, 219; wheatgerm, 220; white, 230; wholemeal, 217. A baguette has 263 calories for the same weight and chapattis made with fat are 328 calories per 100g. Ciabatta is 271 and naan bread averages at 285. A whole white pitta bread is 150 and a wholemeal one is 137, on average.

Don't demonise bread; it's a valuable addition to the diet. The problem with bread is usually what's put on it, rather than the bread itself. However, wholemeal is generally the best choice. It is made with 100 per cent of the grain – the bran and wheatgerm are not present in white bread, and that's where the benefits largely are – high levels of fibre, B vitamins and a whole range of minerals. So white bread has fewer nutrients, despite the fact that white flour has to be fortified with some by law, and it will not keep you feeling as full as wholemeal because it has a higher GI. Check the packaging of commercial loaves because they sometimes have additions like caramel (and even bleach) and may be high in salt. Most bread is low in fat, but watch things like croissants and some speciality breads.

Bread rolls

As rolls vary in size, the calories here are per 100g; weigh them, at least at first. Crusty brown roll, 255, and soft brown, 236; crusty white, 262, and soft white, 254; granary, 238; wholemeal, 244.

As with bread, go for wholemeal to get the full range of benefits. Do watch what is spread on rolls as well as what goes inside.

Bread sticks

A single plain breadstick is, on average, 20 calories.

These are usually made with white flour. If you can stick to a single one, fine – but eating more is all too easy.

Breakfast cereals

A generous helping of most breakfast cereals weighs 35g, and these figures are for that amount: All Bran, 95 calories; branflakes, 116; cornflakes, 132; Oatbran flakes with raisins, 121; Rice Krispies, 134. Muesli is 128 cals, on average, for 50g; two Shredded Wheat have 150 calories and two Weetabix, 127.

What you put on your cereal makes a big difference, as does portion control. Many cereals have high levels of sugar and salt, and it's not always obvious – check packaging once again. They also often have added vitamins and minerals, but do try to avoid the varieties that are high in salt and sugar. Go for ones with lower GI levels, which are made with oats (these have other benefits as well, helping to lower blood cholesterol) or lots of fibre. Sugar-free muesli is a good choice, but be aware that you will need a larger portion size as it's a lot heavier than cereals like cornflakes.

see also OATMEAL, PORRIDGE

Brie
see CHEESE

Broad beans
68 cals/100g.
Broad beans are great. They contain high levels of both soluble and insoluble fibre, protein, carbs, a wide range of vitamins and minerals (including significant amounts of phosphorus for healthy teeth and bones) and quercetin, an antioxidant flavonoid.

Broccoli
A generous helping of florets is 100g – 33 calories.
All members of the Cruciferae group of vegetables – cabbages, kale and the like – are healthy, but broccoli is probably the best. It has more vitamin C than the others, is high in fibre, beta-carotene, folate, potassium, iron … The star benefits, though, come from phytochemicals. The antioxidant lutein maintains healthy eyes and vision, and the Cruciferae contain glucosinolates which help to stimulate the body's natural cancer defences.

Brussels sprouts
42 cals/100g.
These are one of the Cruciferae, like broccoli and cabbage. They're good for fibre, beta-carotene, folate and vitamin C, as well as the phytochemicals. Brussels sprouts are a particularly good source of sinigrin, one of the glucosinolates, which is thought to restrict the growth of pre-cancerous cells.

Buns, etc.
Check packaging carefully, but here are some general guidelines. The average crumpet is 71 calories and an English muffin, 192. American-

style muffins vary hugely and can be as high as 450, so be very wary.
Scones are better as long as they don't come with lots of butter, jam and
cream: a plain white scone, 175; white fruit scone, 150; wholemeal, 116.
Do be careful with these, as even the lower-calorie buns, like crumpets,
are served with very high-calorie additions (can anyone really enjoy
crumpets without lots of butter?).

Burgers
see BEEF

Butter
Weigh butter whenever possible; errors make a big difference as it has 744
calories to 100g. Allow 40 calories for a level teaspoon, roughly what
would go on a slice of toast.
It's not just the calories with butter; it's the saturated fat too – and it's
often high in salt. In butter's favour is the fact that it naturally contains
vitamins A and D, which have to be added to butter substitutes. The
alternatives also contain other ingredients to make them appetising, like
colourings and preservatives. If you decide to continue eating butter,
keep count of how much you use.
See also SPREADS AND MARGARINES

Cabbage
26 cals/100g; red cabbage, 24.
All cabbages are great sources of minerals and vitamins; green cabbage
has more fibre than red. As with other crucifers, the phytochemicals
cabbages contain are particularly important – they are similar to those
found in broccoli. Don't overboil cabbage; try microwaving it to reduce
vitamin loss. Or eat it raw in salads.

Cakes, large and small
Be careful to read packaging; these are best avoided except as special
treats. A medium-sized rich fruit cake can easily contain 5,000 calories
and a slice could be 416 to 625, depending on how generously it is cut;
gâteaux are a minefield. Here are some small cakes: Chelsea bun (75g),

276; custard tart (100g), 277; mince pie (60g), 235; jam doughnuts (75g), 252; ring doughnuts (60g), 242.

Cakes can be a real danger area and the rule is, the plainer the better. Icing, marzipan: not good if you're on a diet of any kind. Watch out for pastry as well – custard tart isn't just high in calories because of the sweet filling.

Camembert

see CHEESE

Carrots

Old carrots are 35 cals/100g; young ones, 30.

Carrots are the richest source of beta-carotene, the precursor of vitamin A and a protective antioxidant. There are actually more nutrients available for the body to use in cooked carrots, because cooking breaks down the thick cell walls. Some fat is necessary to enable the body to absorb it, so it's a good idea to cook carrot soup with a little olive oil, for example. Carrots are a good source of fibre, too, and raw carrot sticks make a healthy nibble.

Cashew nuts

611 cals/100g, and about 15 per nut.

Like all nuts, cashews have significant nutrients: zinc, iron, magnesium, protein and fat. They're quite high in selenium, a useful source of B vitamins and great for vitamin E, but both that and thiamin (vitamin B1) are largely destroyed when the nuts are roasted. A few plain cashew nuts make a great addition to stir-fries.

Cassava

120 cals/100g.

Cassava is mostly starchy carb; it contains very little protein. It does have small quantities of some minerals – potassium, phosphorus, magnesium, iron and selenium – and is a source of vitamin C. Vitamin A and some B vitamins are also present in small quantities.

Cauliflower

34 cals/100g.

Cauliflower is another of the crucifers, like broccoli and cabbage; it is also a good source of valuable glucosinolates which help the body fight damage. It's high in fibre and folate and 100g of raw cauliflower provides more than the recommended daily amount of vitamin C. Cook it in the microwave to retain more of the nutrients.

Celeriac

20 cals/100g.

This swollen root vegetable is a good source of soluble fibre and has useful quantities of folate and potassium – and of vitamin C, when raw. Grated, it makes a delicious salad.

Celery

7 cals/100g; allow 2 per large stick.

There is a substance in celery that may help lower blood pressure and cholesterol levels; research is ongoing. It's also a good source of potassium, which helps maintain healthy blood pressure – but don't dip it in salt.

Cereal bars

These are very variable, so always read the packaging. Don't be fooled into thinking they're always good for you, and check out the ingredients as well as the calories. An average chewy bar has 419 calories per 100g; a crunchy one, 468. Try to find another snack that is better for you, and never use them as an alternative to breakfast.

Cereals

see BREAKFAST CEREALS

Cheese

Always, always weigh cheese until you are used to the size of a smaller portion, perhaps 25g. A convenient eighth of a Camembert is 85 calories, though. These figures are all per 100g: Brie, 343; Cheddar, 416; Cheshire; 371; Edam, 341; Feta, 250; Parmesan, 415; Stilton, 410; Wensleydale, 380.

Cottage cheese has 101 calories per 100g; the low-fat version 79.

Cheese is a good source of protein, a fantastic source of calcium and is useful for the vitamin B12 it contains. Many varieties are also high in salt, fat, calories … However, not all cheeses are the same. As a broad generalisation, hard cheeses (like Parmesan or Cheddar) have the most fat, softer cheeses (Brie, Camembert, Feta) have less and those like ricotta and cottage cheese have the least. Diet versions of some are available, but are often disappointing.

Cherries

48 cals/100g; glacé cherries, 251.

Fresh cherries are wonderful. They contain lots of vitamin C, plenty of potassium and bioflavonoids. Glacé cherries, though, are very, very high in sugar.

Cheshire cheese

see CHEESE

Chestnuts

170 cals/100g.

Chestnuts are different from other nuts. They are high in complex carbohydrates, with very little protein or fat by comparison, and have a higher water content – which is why they have fewer calories. They are good for fibre, vitamins E and B6, and potassium.

Chicken

Chicken meat has an average of 107 cals/100g raw weight, and a skinless boned chicken breast is about 120g – 128 calories. Roast chicken on a rack, so fat can drain away.

Chicken is a great source of protein. It is only low in fat if the skin is removed because chicken skin is very high in calories and saturated fat. Chicken meat is a good source of B vitamins and selenium. Dark meat has twice the zinc and iron of white meat but that contains more phosphorus and potassium – so eat both. Ready-made poultry products are usually highly processed and contain lots of additives.

Chickpeas
Dried, 320 cals/100g; canned and drained, 115.
Chickpeas are a great source of fibre and have all the benefits of beans, but they are also especially good sources of vitamin E and manganese. They have useful amounts of iron and folate, too. And a lovely nutty taste!

Chicory and radicchio
11 cals/100g.
These contain some vitamin C, folate and thiamin. Radicchio's red colour is a sign of beta-carotene, and darker leaves contain more than pale ones. It has a higher level of vitamin C than chicory.

Chillies
20 cals/100g, but no one would use that much normally. Their calories are negligible in most dishes.
Be careful handling fresh chillies – don't rub your eyes or nose, and wash your hands when you've finished. The distinctive substance they contain, capsaicin, provides a lot of heat, but it's also a powerful antioxidant with anti-inflammatory effects. Chillies are also a good source of vitamin C.

Chinese leaves (also known as Chinese cabbage)
28 cals/100g
Chinese leaves are a good source of protective glucosinolates, like broccoli and other cruciferous plants, but don't have as much as those with darker leaves. They also contain folate, vitamin C and potassium.

Chips
see POTATOES

Chocolate
Milk chocolate, 520 cals/100g; plain, 510; white, 529. Fruit and nut, 550; whole nut, 490.

Chocolate is high in fat, but that's not the whole story. Weighed (and in moderation), it's a permissible snack – especially chocolate with over 70 per cent cocoa solids, which may have antioxidant benefits. All chocolate contains an amount of sugar (which varies widely), some protein, caffeine and potassium; milk chocolate has useful amounts of calcium and plain is more than twice as high in iron and magnesium.

Chutney and pickles

Per tablespoon of average chutney (20g): 38; sweet pickle, 28; piccalilli, 17; mango chutney, 60; brinjal pickle, 74. A cocktail onion has only 1 calorie and large pickled onions have an average of 10 each. Gherkins and cornichons have 14 cals/100g – that's a lot, if they are small or medium in size.

Go easy with most chutneys – whether they're traditional British ones, like a sweet pickle or those with an Indian influence – as they may contain a lot of sugar and the calories can mount up. Pickles can be high in salt, but are often a better choice. Most pickled fruit or vegetables retain some of their mineral content, though vitamins are usually destroyed in the pickling process.

see also SAUERKRAUT

Cider

For half a pint (275 ml), dry cider has 99 calories, sweet has 116, vintage has 278; low-alcohol cider has only 47.

Cider is higher in potassium than beer, but it's a negligible quantity really. It doesn't have many nutritional virtues.

Clementines

see ORANGES, ETC.

Cockles

Boiled, 53 cals/100g.

Cockles are a good source of vitamin B12, iron, iodine and selenium. Don't, however, collect them from the shore yourself unless you are certain the water is unpolluted – check with the local council if in doubt.

Cocoa and drinking chocolate

Cocoa and chocolate powders are high in calories, but you don't use that much – check packaging information for calorie values, as they vary a lot. Bear in mind that what you make them up with will affect calorie values and opt for skimmed milk. Both cocoa and chocolate powder contain flavonoids with antioxidant properties, but they can be very high in fat indeed. Calcium will come from the milk, too, and hot chocolate contains vitamins B2 and B12.

Coconut

Desiccated coconut has 604 cals/100g; creamed coconut in a block is 669 per 100g. Coconut milk, tinned, has 240 calories per 100g and the lower-fat version is 105. Fresh coconut milk has 22.

Coconut – and its derivatives – is high in saturated fat. It might not be as harmful as the kind found in animal products, but research to establish this is still in progress. It's also a good source of potassium. Raw coconut does contain fibre, but all round coconut is poor in nutrients when compared to other nuts. Its taste, however, is a different matter – but do use it in moderation.

Cod

Raw cod fillet has 80 calories per 100g; when cooked in batter that figure rises to 247. Hard roe, coated in breadcrumbs and fried, is 202 per 100g.

Cod is high in protein, low in fat and a great source of B group vitamins as well as some minerals – particularly iodine, selenium and potassium. Chip-shop cod is just too high in calories, though, and can really blow a diet.

Coffee

2 cals/100ml. That's without milk or sugar. Beware of a lot of the cappuccino mixes; they are often high in calories and saturated fats.

Coffee gets a varied response from experts: some say a little may do you good and others think you should cut it out completely, largely because of the caffeine it contains. It's a complicated substance, with 300 other active ingredients as well. Some are antioxidants, and there's one vitamin – niacin.

Cognac
see LIQUEURS

Coleslaw
see SALADS, READY-MADE

Cooking fats
Beef dripping has 891 cals/100g, as has lard; ghee has 898.
These are all high in saturated fats as well as calories, so measure carefully and think about using a healthier oil instead. It should not be too difficult to change, and doing so could really benefit your health (and your diet).
see also OILS, SUET

Cooking sauces
Many are high in calories – they may look reasonable per 100g or 100ml but you'll use at least double that quantity. Levels of additives, sugar and salt can also be high. It is best to avoid them, or make your own so you can control the ingredients.

Cornflour
354 cals/100g; a level tablespoon is 53.
This is generally used in small quantities as a thickener. It's high in starch, low in fat, without useful quantities of minerals and only trace quantities of vitamins.

Cornish pasty
These are variable, but the average pasty is about 200g – and they have 267 calories per 100g.

Pasties are often high in saturated fats and trans fats. They sometimes have good-quality minerals, but vitamin content is not brilliant. They are likely to be processed – with many ingredients you wouldn't find in the average kitchen – and are worth avoiding.

Corn-on-the-cob

see SWEETCORN

Cottage cheese

see CHEESE

Courgette and marrow

Courgettes have 18 cals/100g; marrows, 12.

Courgettes are low in fat and a good source of beta-carotene; they also contain vitamin C and folate. There are few nutritional goodies in marrow, though – it's 95 per cent water, with minimal beta-carotene. It's not even high in fibre; courgettes have more of that by weight, too.

Cous cous

355 cals/100g, dry weight; the average helping is 50g.

The nutritional value of couscous depends on what type it is. Most is now pre-cooked; you only need to steam it and serve. It's low in fat, and that's about it. Traditional couscous, the type you might find in a health-food shop, takes longer to cook but has more nutrients.

Crab

Fresh crab, white and dark meat, is 128 cals/100g. Crabsticks have 68.

Fresh crab is a good source of protein and has significant quantities of omega-3 fatty acids. It also has great levels of riboflavin, potassium and zinc, as well as vitamin B6 and magnesium. Crabsticks, however, are actually made of minced fish – go for unprocessed crab or fish instead.

Crackers and crispbreads

These vary, but labelling is usually clear. A cream cracker is 29, as is a wholemeal cracker; matzo crackers are 19 each. Crispbreads can range from being very low (9 calories) to a lot higher (54) per biscuit, depending on additional ingredients (such as cheese).

Some crackers could add fibre to your diet; others might not. Use the pack information to help you judge, and double-check salt and sugar levels.

see also OATCAKES, RICE CAKES

Cranberries

Fresh, 16 cals/100g. Dried ones have 360, and also often have sugar or apple juice added.

Cranberries have often been called a 'superfood'. They are a great source of antioxidants, vitamins C and D, potassium and iron. However, they are sour and generally need sweetening – bear that in mind when you're calorie counting. They're often used to fight infections, particularly those of the urinary tract, and their effectiveness has been supported by scientific research.

see also FRUIT AND VEGETABLE JUICES

Cream

Single cream has 193 cals/100 ml; double, 496; clotted 586; whipping, 381. Crème fraîche has 378.

Cream is high in fat, often saturated, so use it sparingly. It is a useful source of vitamin A, but so are many other more healthy foods (such as eggs, fish oil and liver). There are reduced-fat creams available, though some are more successful than others. Try yoghurt as an alternative, or even a soya 'cream': it's not as unappealing as you might think.

Crisps and savoury snacks

The average 34.5g bag of crisps has 183 calories, about 530 per 100g. Many snacks of this type come in differently sized packs, so here are some comparisons by 100g: Bombay mix, 503; mini popadums, 515; potato rings, 523; Pringles original, 540; tortilla chips, average, 459; Twiglets, 383. 'Hand-cooked' crisps are lower, at an average 480 per 100g, but they are heavier so you don't get so many for 100g.

These are all high in salt and fat (not as much saturated fat as they used to have, but they're still no health food) and have very few nutritional benefits. It might be easier to cut them out completely than to try and cut down.

Croissants

The size of these varies but the average medium croissant has 200 or more calories.

Croissants do contain folate, but they also have high saturated fat levels – they're made with butter, after all. Don't add even more.

Crumpets

see BUNS

Cucumber

10 cals/100g.

Cucumber skin contains beta-carotene as well as plant sterols, which may help lower blood cholesterol levels. Otherwise, cucumbers have few elements with nutritional value – they're 96.4 per cent water.

Currants

see SULTANAS, CURRANTS AND RAISINS

Curry

There is a huge range of curries available in shops and restaurants and many are high in calories.

As a rule of thumb, choose something plain like a simple tandoori rather than a creamy korma, and watch out for coconut milk in Thai curries, which pushes their calorie values up.

Custard

This changes according to how you make it. Made with full-cream milk, it has 118 calories per 100g; with semi-skimmed that goes down to 95. It is also higher in saturated fat when you use whole milk. Ready-to-eat custard – 98 cals/100g – has none and is lower in most other nutrients too. It can be high in additives, so check packaging for details.

....

Damsons

see PLUMS

....

Dandelions and wild leaves

These are increasingly popular additions to salads, and very low in calories. Allow 20 calories per 100g, but you are not likely to use that much. Don't pick them from polluted sites, and always rinse them.

Dandelions contain beta-carotene, calcium, potassium and more iron than spinach. Nettles are high in beta-carotene too, as well as vitamin C, calcium, potassium and iron. Discard the stalks of young nettles, rinse the leaves – and make a great soup, or brew some nettle tea. Sorrel is high in beta-carotene and vitamin C, but also contains oxalic acid. This can slow the absorption of iron and calcium, so use it with moderation. Sorrel sauce is good with oily fish, and young leaves of wild garlic are delicious in most salads.

....

Dates

Dried dates have 270 calories per 100g; a single medium date is about 10g – 27 calories. Fresh dates are 124 calories per 100g.

Fresh dates are better for vitamin C, but both are good sources of fibre. Dried dates contain more sugar than fresh ones, but they're also richer in potassium and a more concentrated source of niacin, iron, copper and magnesium.

....

Deli meats

see MEATS, COLD AND DELI

....

Dips

Comparison is best done by 100g; though the pots sold in supermarkets are usually 200g, they do vary. Guacamole, 210 cals/100g; hummus, average (shop bought), 315; 'low-fat' hummus, 185; taramasalata, 504; tsatsiki, 66. Dips based on sour cream can be very high so read packs carefully – they average about 400 calories per 100g. Tomato salsa, by contrast, has 49.

Some dips are better for you than others, but generally approach ready-made dips with caution. Taramasalata, for example, has plenty of vitamin B12, but is high in fat and salt. Hummus, the chickpea and tahini dip, is best home-made; fortunately it's very easy. Most commercial versions don't contain as many chickpeas, and the home-made version is a better source of nutrients.

Dressings

see SALAD DRESSINGS

Drinks

see BEERS, CIDER, LIQUEURS, PORT, SHERRY, SPIRITS, VERMOUTH, WINE; FRUIT AND VEGETABLE JUICES; FRUIT SMOOTHIES; FRUIT SQUASHES; FIZZY DRINKS; MIXERS; TEA; COFFEE

Duck

The skin pushes the calories up, as it does for all poultry; it increases the saturated fat content, too. Roast duck, meat only, is 195 cals/100g; with skin, that figure rises to 423. Raw, there are 137 calories in 100g of duck, without skin.

Duck is a good source of all B vitamins; in fact, it is higher in B vitamins, selenium and zinc than chicken. It has more than three times the amount of iron, too, as well as being a source of potassium. It is, however, higher in fat and calories than chicken.

Edam

see CHEESE

Eel (jellied)

98 cals/100g

This is low in fat, and most of it is monounsaturated. It is a good source of selenium and vitamin E, though it is also quite salty. You can also buy non-jellied eel, which can be a better choice.

Eggs

A small hen's egg has 70 calories, a medium one 85, and a large one 100. Egg yolk, per 100g, has 339 calories and egg white, 36. This is almost negligible, really, because 100g of egg white is quite a lot.

Eggs are a nutritional powerhouse, so don't abandon them because you're worried about cholesterol – cholesterol from food has been shown to have little or no effect on blood cholesterol levels. Eggs are a fantastic source of protein, the right fats, vitamin B12 and a whole host of minerals. Hens are sometimes fed special supplements to boost particular nutrients, like omega-3 fatty acids. In general, there are more nutrients in organic eggs, so go for these if at all possible and cook them so you add as few calories as possible – boiling or poaching rather than scrambling or frying.

Elderberries

73 cals/100g.

It is worth gathering elderberries as they are very high in vitamin C, vitamin A and potassium – just make sure you collect them somewhere away from traffic and any other sources of pollution. They will need some sugar or fructose added during cooking to make them palatable.

Endive

16 cals/100g.

Endive is a good addition to salads; it's a useful source of thiamin and vitamin C and contains almost twice the fibre of lettuce. It has an interesting taste, too.

Falafel

These vary, but average 53 calories per falafel.

If you fry them, you will add a lot more calories. Commercial brands are generally made from chickpeas and have some of their benefits, including fibre, vitamin E and manganese. Serve with a mixed salad; there's no need to stuff them in pitta bread with dollops of hummus and tsatsiki.

Fats,

see COOKING FATS, OILS

Fennel

12 cals/100g.

The bulbous root of Florence fennel is a source of beta-carotene, folate and potassium, and a crunchy addition to salads. It also has good levels of fibre.

Feta

see CHEESE

Figs

37 calories per fresh fig; dried figs are 227 per 100g.

Dried figs are high in fibre and potassium, but also in sugar. They're a concentrated source of calcium, iron, magnesium, zinc and vitamin B6. Fresh figs contain some fibre – always eat the skin – and have useful quantities of beta-carotene as well as vitamin B6.

Fish

see ANCHOVIES, COD, EEL, HADDOCK, HALIBUT, HERRING, KIPPER, LEMON SOLE, MACKEREL, MONKFISH, PILCHARDS, PLAICE, RED MULLET, SALMON, SARDINES, SEA BASS, SKATE, SMOKED FISH, SWORDFISH, TROUT, TUNA, WHITEBAIT

Fish fingers

They average 50 calories for a grilled fish finger.

Don't fry them as that would require extra fat and they are just as easily cooked under the grill. They are a source of B vitamins and several minerals, including iodine and selenium.

Fizzy drinks

When reading labels, bear in mind that a can usually contains 330ml, and the calories are often only given for 100ml. A can of cola can vary

between 136 calories and none, depending on the type; ginger ale is 50 for a can; lemonade averages at 73. 'Energy' drinks are often higher, containing high levels of glucose.

Many fizzy drinks have lots of sugar or artificial sweeteners and some are high in caffeine; they have even been linked to an accelerated risk of bone loss. At any rate, they have few nutritional benefits and are worth abandoning. At the very least, switch to diet versions but watch out for those artificial sweeteners.

Flapjacks

see BISCUITS

Flour

All figures are for 100g. White wheat flour, 341; wholemeal wheat flour, 310; spelt, 311, rye, 335. Gram flour, which is made from chickpeas, has 313.

Wholemeal flour is better than refined white flour. It contains more nutrients: more protein, three times as much fibre, greater quantities of many minerals and vitamins. White flour, though, contains more calcium, and has to be fortified with some nutrients by law. Rye flour has great vitamin and mineral levels, though it often needs to be mixed with wheat flour as it's low in gluten, and is even higher in fibre than wholemeal. Spelt is more nutritious than many modern strains of wheat and the gluten it contains is a different type, which some people find easier to digest, so give spelt flour a try. Gram flour has many of the benefits of chickpeas.

French beans

see GREEN BEANS

Fromage frais

The little pots are usually 50g. A plain one averages 57 calories, a fruit one 62; some may be higher, so check.

They are a good source of calcium, but the saturated fat content can be quite high. Watch out for artificial ingredients in flavoured ones.

Fruit

see ACKEE, APPLES, APRICOTS, AVOCADO, BANANAS, BLACKBERRIES, BLACKCURRANTS AND REDCURRANTS, BLUEBERRIES AND BILBERRIES, CHERRIES, CRANBERRIES, DATES, ELDERBERRIES, FIGS, GOOSEBERRIES, GRAPEFRUIT, GRAPES, GUAVAS, KIWI FRUIT, LEMON, LIMES, LYCHEES, MANGOES, MELON, NECTARINE, ORANGES ETC., PAPAYA, PASSION FRUIT, PEACHES, PEARS, PINEAPPLE, PLUMS, POMEGRANATE, RASPBERRIES, RHUBARB, SHARON FRUIT AND PERSIMMONS, STRAWBERRIES; SULTANAS, CURRANTS AND RAISINS; TOMATOES, WATERMELON

Fruit and vegetable juices

Apple, 38 cals/100ml; cranberry, 61; grape, 46; grapefruit, 33; pineapple, 41; pomegranate, 44 cals; orange, 36. Carrot has 24 and tomato juice, 14. Most large glasses contain 250–300ml.

All fruit juices are high in vitamin C, though it may be added to commerically prepared apple juice because apples have lower levels than some other fruits. All juices are lacking in fibre. When it comes to orange juice, go for freshly squeezed: it retains more flavonoids. Grapefruit juice can affect the performance of some prescription drugs – be aware of that and check with your doctor if you take medication. Tomato juice contains lycopene, an antioxidant. Bear in mind that fruit juice only counts as one portion of your five a day, no matter how much you drink. And if you have a smoothie as well, that does not count as a second portion.

Fruit smoothies

Smoothies are much healthier than fruit squashes (see below). They have a higher proportion of fruit and some fibre, as well as nutrients from any milk or yoghurt they contain. Their calorie content depends on ingredients, so check packaging or make your own by liquidising fruit with yoghurt or milk; commercial ones may well also contain colouring and preservatives. As a basic rule, smoothies average about 50–60 calories per 100ml. Like fruit juices, smoothies only count as a single portion of the five-a-day aim for fruit and vegetables, even if you have more than one.

Fruit squashes

Many fruit squashes are almost pure sugar before dilution and it's better to use an alternative: sugar quantity can range from one teaspoon of sugar per 200ml glass to a staggering four. They also generally contain very little real fruit juice – and do not count towards the five-a-day target at all.

Game

Roast pheasant (meat only) is 220 cals/100g; pigeon has 208 and grouse 144. Roast venison has 165. Rabbit is 132 cals/100g, raw weight; allow 381 cals/100g for game pie.

All game is a source of B vitamins and some minerals, especially iron and potassium. It is often a comparatively low-fat source of protein. Game pie is not; the pastry undoes all the benefits of the lower levels of fat in the meat.

Garlic

One clove has 2 calories.

From a dieting point of view, garlic adds lots of flavour at minimal calorie cost. The antioxidants it contains can help to prevent blood clots from forming (which can cause heart attacks and stroke) – but they are destroyed if you cook it for longer than about five minutes. Crushing breaks down the cell walls and makes these nutrients more readily available. There's some scientific support for the idea that garlic stimulates the immune system and acts as an antibacterial agent, and it's even been said that people who eat it regularly are less prone to cancer.

Gherkins and cornichons

see CHUTNEY AND PICKLES

Ginger

A 2-cm piece has 2 calories.

Like garlic, this adds flavour without adding lots of calories. It's also often used to combat nausea and colds, and as an aid to digestion.

Grate it in stir fries for an Eastern flavour, or add some to fresh juices (it works well with carrot, apple or pear).

Ginger ale

see FIZZY DRINKS, MIXERS

Goose

Roasted, meat and skin, 310 cals/100g.

Goose is quite a fatty meat, and it's worth avoiding the skin; roast it on a rack to drain off as much fat as possible. It contains more riboflavin (B2) than chicken and about twice the vitamin B6, and is a good source of potassium, phosphorus and iron. Goose fat can add a lot of saturated fat to roast potatoes, so don't cook them in it.

Gooseberries

19 cals/100g, raw. Stewed with sugar, they can be about 55 – it depends on the quantity of sugar.

Both fresh and cooked gooseberries are a useful source of soluble fibre and vitamin C; only a little is lost in the cooking. They are sometimes really sour, though, so be careful about adding sugar (taste them first to check how much they need) and watch cream too – gooseberry fool is gorgeous, but not at all slimming.

Grains

All figures are for 100g. Buckwheat, roasted, 378; bulgur wheat, 357; millet, 384; semolina, 350; wheat bran, 206; wheatgerm, 357. Pot barley is 302 and pearl barley 360 calories.

Most grains are complex carbohydrates, high in fibre, so they are good low-GI additions to the diet. Many are also high in B vitamins and minerals. Refined versions – like pearl barley – have less fibre and fewer nutritional benefits.

see also COUSCOUS, OATMEAL, POLENTA, QUINOA

Gram flour

see FLOUR

Grapefruit

30 cals/100g – an average half.

All grapefruit is high in vitamin C and contains valuable bioflavonoids, and the pink version also has useful amounts of beta-carotene. Grapefruit can interact with certain prescription drugs, so talk to your doctor if you are taking, for example, statins, AIDS drugs or antidepressants. Finally, the grapefruit diet was once popular and still resurfaces; it's supposed to help you 'burn fat'. It doesn't. It can, however, make you ill because it doesn't contain enough nutrients to sustain life.

Grapes

60 cals/100g.

Grapes are a good source of potassium, but don't contain a lot of vitamin C compared to other fruit. Red and black grapes are higher in important antioxidants.

Gravy

Instant gravy, made up following pack instructions, has 34 calories per 100ml, though it's usually high in salt.

Gravy made from meat juices can be very high in fat; skim the excess fat off the juices first, as that will help.

Green or French beans

24 cals/100g.

These are a great source of fibre and also have useful quantities of beta-carotene, folate, vitamin C, vitamin K, potassium and calcium. Don't overboil them – in fact, try them raw in salads.

Greengages

see PLUMS

Grouse

see GAME

Guacamole

see DIPS

....

Guavas

26 cals/100g raw; tinned, in syrup: 60.

Fresh guavas are a fantastic source of vitamin C (they have more than five times that in an orange, weight for weight), and a good one for potassium and fibre. Only about 25 per cent of the vitamin C is lost in the canning process, but do watch out for sugary syrups and drain canned guava well.

....

Haddock

Raw weight, 81 cals/100g; steamed, 89. Steamed smoked haddock has 101 cals/100g.

A great low-fat source of protein, unless it's coated in batter and deep-fried. Haddock is high in the B vitamins, especially B6 and B12, potassium, selenium and iodine. Smoked haddock can be high in sodium, so avoid it if high blood pressure is a problem.

see also SMOKED FISH

....

Halibut

116 cals/100g, raw weight.

A white fish, halibut is high in protein, potassium, vitamin A, the B vitamins (particularly niacin), iodine, potassium and phosphorus.

....

Ham and gammon

Cold ham averages 107 cals/100g; wafer-thin ham is 108. Parma ham is much higher, at 248, but you get a lot for 100g. A gammon joint, raw weight, has 138 cals/100g; grilled gammon rashers have 199.

Like bacon, ham and gammon are high in salt because of the way they are cured. Extra-lean ham is a good source of relatively low-fat protein and, like all meat, is also high in many B vitamins and potassium. Canned ham, though, only really has useful levels of B1, and Parma ham is very fatty. Gammon is a good source of vitamins B1 and B6, potassium, phosphorus and zinc.

Hazelnuts

650 cals/100g; 10g is about 8 or 9 nuts – 65 calories.

Hazelnuts are high in monounsaturated fats and essential fatty acids. They are also a great source of other nutrients: vitamins B1, B6, niacin, folate and E as well as many minerals. Vitamin E is largely destroyed by roasting, though.

Herbs

The calories in herbs are negligible – forget about it and use them wherever you wish. Their nutritional value is also generally low, simply because of the small quantities that are used, but they are fantastic for seasoning and flavouring food. Parsley is often used in greater quantities and contains beta-carotene, vitamins C and E as well as folate and various phytochemicals. For the full range of nutritional benefits, fresh is better than dried.

Herring

Raw weight, 190 cals/100g. A large rollmop has about 110 calories.

One of the oily fish, high in omega-3 fatty acids as well as in monounsaturated fats. Herring is also high in B vitamins, vitamin D (it's much better than the other oily fish for this), phosphorus, selenium, iodine, zinc and potassium. The only really significant vitamin in pickled herring is B6.

see also KIPPERS

Honey

288 cals/100g and about 25 per teaspoon.

Honey has negligible amounts of nutrients other than simple carbs – slightly better than white sugar, which has none – but it's unlikely to be eaten in sufficient quantities to reap any particular benefits. It does, however, have antiseptic properties. It often has an interesting flavour, which depends on the flowers the bees have visited.

Hummus

see DIPS

Ice cream and frozen desserts

There is an enormous variation in calorie values here, so always check packaging; some luxury brands of ice cream can be very high. Fruit sorbet is generally the best option and, when it comes to individual ices, sorbet lollipops are the ones to pick. Most commercial frozen desserts are high in sugar, artificial ingredients and often in fat – sometimes from rather surprising sources (vegetarians should check labels carefully). Milk-based desserts have some calcium from the milk, and most varieties of ice cream contain vitamins A, B2 and B12.

Jam

Allow about 20 cals for a level teaspoonful.

High in sugar, low in other nutrients: there are tiny amounts of some vitamins and the fruit in jam makes a minimal contribution to fibre levels. Cheaper brands may use artificial colouring and have a higher proportion of sugar to fruit.

Jelly

A block of jelly has 296 cals/100g and weighs, generally, 135g – 400 calories. It serves four when made up and a ready-to-eat jelly pot for children has 100 calories. Reduced-sugar jelly powders are available; their calories are usually very low.

Jelly is mostly water and carbohydrate – and simple carbs, at that – with some protein. There are small quantities of some minerals, but no vitamins; nor is there any truth in the old story that the gelatine it contains strengthens nails.

Juices

see FRUIT AND VEGETABLE JUICES

Kale

33 cals/100g.

Kale is often called a superfood because of the wide range of useful phytochemicals it contains. It's an excellent source of beta-carotene, vitamins C and E – all of them antioxidants – and also of glucosinolates, like the rest of the crucifers (*see* BROCCOLI). It contains folate as well, and is a good source of calcium, potassium, manganese and iron.

Kidneys

see OFFAL

Kipper

229 cals/100g.

Kippers, cured herrings, are high in good fats and protein and also provide B vitamins, vitamin D and a range of minerals. Salt content can be high because of the way they are cured, and try to avoid ones coloured with synthetic dyes.

see also SMOKED FISH

Kiwi fruit

49 cals/100g, and the average kiwi is about 80g – 39 calories.

Kiwi fruit are a fantastic source of vitamin C. They're also high in vitamin E and potassium, but do have less fibre overall than some fruit. Soluble fibre levels are fine, though.

Kohlrabi

23 cals/100g.

A good source of vitamin C, potassium and both kinds of fibre. It doesn't have a particularly strong taste, but makes a crunchy addition to salads.

Lager

see BEERS

Lamb

Raw weight, trimmed of excess fat, 153 cals/100g; cutlets are 316 cals/100g, and lamb mince has 196. Lean roast lamb has 203 calories to 100g.

The amount of saturated fat in lamb is very variable, depending on factors like the breed of sheep it comes from and the time of year. Some joints are much fattier than others – shoulder, for example. Leg is the leanest. Always trim off visible fat before cooking. Lamb is a good source of protein, B vitamins, iron and zinc.

Lard

see COOKING FATS

Leeks

22 cals/100g.
Leeks contain similar antioxidants to onions and related vegetables which appear to stimulate the immune system. They are useful for the potassium and folate they contain, and also have beta-carotene, vitamin C and potassium.

Lemon

Don't bother too much about the calories in lemons unless you are using a lot – they have 19 cals/100g, juice and skin, and that's about a medium to large lemon. Lemon juice by itself is only 7 cals/100ml.
Lemons are a good source of vitamin C and can enhance the flavour of other foods; they also have similar phytochemicals to other citrus fruits. Do buy organic ones, though, as pesticides can penetrate the peel to some degree.

Lemon sole

Raw weight, 83 cals/100g. Sole goujons are much worse – baked, coated ones are 187, and fried ones rise to 374.
It's worth avoiding sole goujons, but the fish itself is a great low-fat source of protein. It also has B vitamins, especially niacin, as well as good levels of magnesium, potassium and selenium.

Lentils

Green and brown lentils have 297 cals/100g, dry weight. Dry red lentils have 318. A hundred grams of boiled lentils is 100 calories.

Lentils have many of the same benefits as beans. Green and brown lentils have lots of fibre (both soluble and insoluble), protein, a range of B vitamins and selenium. They're also a useful source of iron and manganese, phosphorus, zinc, copper, potassium … Red lentils, which have no skins, are less nutritious and have about half the quantity of fibre, but it's still plenty.

Lettuces and salad leaves

You can forget about counting calories for lettuce and salad leaves – a dessert bowl is roughly 60g and 8 calories.

But you can't forget about dressings, or about items like croûtons that might be included in a pre-packed bag of salad. They can be very high in calories. The nutritional content of salad leaves varies according to the level of freshness and the time of year, but in general darker leaves are a much better source of nutrients than pale ones, so a cos is a better choice than an iceberg lettuce. They're high in beta-carotene and can also be a useful source of folate and potassium.

see also ENDIVE, DANDELION AND WILD LEAVES

Limes

A single lime – juice and skin – is only 3 calories.

A good source of vitamin C, and with significant bioflavonoids (like other citrus fruit), limes are an excellent flavouring to use.

Linseeds

470 cals/100g; a level teaspoon is 24.

Linseeds are a good source of fibre, omega-3 fatty acids and phytochemicals. But they do need to be ground – whole ones are too tough for the body to digest. They can be sprinkled on cereals or added to smoothies and bread.

Liqueurs

Bear in mind measures – it can be very easy to pour yourself a larger drink at home than you would be served in a bar. Here are some, by

100ml for comparison: Baileys, 320; Cognac, 350; Cointreau, 340; Tia Maria, 260.

Many liqueurs are very sweet and creamy ones like Baileys also contain some fat. The creamy ones may have small amounts of minerals and vitamins, but they are too insignificant to have much nutritional value.

Liver

see OFFAL

Lobster

103 cals/100g, boiled.

Lobster is a good low-fat source of protein. It has excellent levels of vitamin B12 and niacin and good quantities of many minerals including zinc and selenium – it has more selenium than other shellfish. Fatty accompaniments can be a problem, though, so avoid sauces or mayonnaise.

Lychees

Fresh lychees are 58 cals/100g. Tinned ones vary; drained, they can be 68.

Lychees are a source of vitamin C and contain some fibre, but watch out for the sugar content of tinned ones. They make an unusual and refreshing addition to a fruit salad.

Macadamia nuts

748 cals/100g.

Macadamia nuts are higher in fat than other nuts, which pushes up the calories, but it is mostly monounsaturated fat. They are a particularly good source of manganese.

Mackerel

Raw weight, 220 cals/100g; smoked mackerel, 354.

One of the oily fish, mackerel is high in monounsaturated fat and a wonderful source of omega-3 fatty acids. It's also high in B vitamins, vitamin D and several minerals, particularly iodine. Smoked mackerel is high in salt because of the way it is cured, but retains most of the nutritional benefits.

see also SMOKED FISH

Mangetout
32 cals/100g, raw.
Mangetout peas are high in fibre because the pods are eaten and they are a good source of beta-carotene and most minerals, especially potassium. They also have good levels of protein, but less than ordinary peas as the tiny peas inside the pods are immature. The pods do give mangetout a higher level of vitamin C, though.

Mangoes
Fresh, without the stone, 57 cals/100g; dried, 350 cals/100g.
A fantastic source of beta-carotene; mangoes have more than most fruits. They also have high levels of vitamin C and useful quantities of most minerals, particularly potassium and manganese. They're a good source of fibre, especially soluble – but are quite high in sugar.

Maple syrup
see SYRUPS

Margarine
see SPREADS AND MARGARINES

Marmalade
About 20 calories for a level teaspoonful.
Like jam, marmalade does not have much of value other than the sugar it contains. Use it in moderation.

Marmite and Bovril
Marmite is 180 cals/100g; Bovril, 179. In both cases a small teaspoonful, the amount you'd be likely to use on two large slices of toast, is 9 cals.

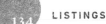

Marmite, like other yeast extracts, is very rich in protein, B vitamins and some minerals. Bovril is also a good source for these. Unfortunately both are high in salt, but they are generally eaten in small quantities.

Marrow

see COURGETTE AND MARROW

Marzipan

389 cals/100g.

Usually made with ground almonds, sugar and egg, marzipan is high in protein, carbohydrates, fat – and therefore in calories. Commercial varieties vary in their nutritional values, but marzipan can contain quite decent quantities of minerals and some vitamins when well made (when it is not, it may be bulked up with sugar rather than almonds, and may not contain any egg).

Mayonnaise

A level tablespoon of extra-light mayo is 15 calories; of light or reduced-calorie mayo, 45; and of a standard one, 105.

There are many 'diet' versions of mayonnaise available, but you may prefer to use less of an ordinary one for the fuller flavour. If you do, be careful. Home-made mayonnaise is rich in vitamin E and uses olive oil, where most commercial brands do not – but it may contain artificial flavourings and colours and is high in calories. Whatever option you go for, do remember to keep tabs on quantities.

see also SALAD DRESSINGS

Meat

see BACON, BEEF, CHICKEN, DUCK, GAME, HAM AND GAMMON, LAMB; MEATS, COLD AND DELI; OFFAL, PORK, SAUSAGES, TURKEY

Meats, cold and deli

Salami averages 490 cals/100g. A thin slice of Milano salami weighs about 6g and has about 20–25 calories, so be careful. Chorizo averages

500 cals/100g; Cervelat is 408. Cold meats like turkey roll are lower –
166 cals/100g; corned beef has 205 and tongue has 289.

Many deli meats are high in fat, frequently saturated. They also have high levels of salt and may have additives like artificial preservatives and colourings. They are best approached with caution when you are trying to diet and eat more healthily; the best choice is simple cold, roast meat with the fat removed.

see also HAM AND GAMMON, SAUSAGES

Melon

Canteloupe melon has 19 cals/100g, galia 24 and honeydew 28.

Nutritionally, melons vary a lot. Canteloupe is amazingly high in beta-carotene; pale-fleshed ones like honeydew contain much less and have less vitamin C. All melons have a high water content, which is why they are comparatively low in calories.

see also WATERMELON

Milk

Here, for comparison, are figures per 100ml; they may not look high
but remember that most tall glasses hold about 250–300ml. Full-
cream milk, 66 cals/100ml; semi-skimmed, 46; skimmed, 32. Channel
Island milk has 78 and 'breakfast' milk has 72. Goats' milk has 62,
and sheep's milk 93. Evaporated milk has 151 calories and sweetened
condensed milk has 333. A 15 ml tablespoon is about the amount that
would normally go in a cup of tea or coffee, but check you don't use
more, and see page 59 for advice on an easy way to assess your daily
milk calories.

Milk contains a wide range of nutrients. It can be very high in saturated fat, so make sure you use skimmed which retains most of the nutrients in full-cream milk without the high fat content (though vitamin A is lost). Milk contains good levels of essential B vitamins, phosphorus and zinc, but the star mineral is calcium. The calcium from milk is easily absorbed by the body, too. Goats' milk is almost as fatty as full-cream cows' milk; sheep's milk is even fattier.

see also SOYA MILK

Milkshake

These vary a lot. An average figure is 88 calories per 100ml, but bear in mind that serving sizes can be much bigger than that.

A large milkshake could come to almost a third of your recommended daily calorie intake, contain a lot of saturated fat and a variety of artificial ingredients.

Mince

see BEEF AND LAMB

Mixers

A small bottle (113ml) of bitter lemon has 40 calories and tonic water has 30; opt for low-calorie versions at 4 and 2 calories respectively. Ginger ale has 43. The small cans of mixers contain 150 ml.

Nutritionally, mixers don't add much – except calories from the sugars they contain. Swap to low-calorie versions.

Monkfish

Raw weight, 70 cals/100g.

A white fish with firm-textured flesh, monkfish is good as a low-fat source of protein and contains a wide range of vitamins and minerals.

Mooli or white radish

15 cals/100g.

Mooli is generally eaten for its crunchiness and its peppery taste when fresh, rather than any nutritional contribution it makes. It's a useful source of vitamin C, and that's about it.

Muffins

see BUNS

Mushrooms

13 cals/100g, raw weight.

All mushrooms have very little carbohydrate compared to the protein and fibre they contain. They are a source of B vitamins, potassium and trace elements like copper; some varieties contain useful phytochemicals. There's little difference, however, between wild and cultivated types and they all soak up fat, so watch how you cook them.

Mussels

Boiled, 104 cals/100g.

Mussels are a great low-fat source of protein, vitamin E, B vitamins including folate and many minerals, and they are particularly high in iron and iodine. Do be careful about the sauces they are served in – avoid high-fat ones, particularly those with cream, and select ones cooked in wine, tomatoes or flavoured stock.

Mustard

Dijon mustard has 30 calories per tablespoon, English mustard has 40. In practice you would probably use about a third of that.

Because mustard isn't generally used in large quantities, its impact on the overall diet is low. It does, however, have a range of minerals so it's worth adding to salad dressings or serving with meat.

Mustard and cress

13 cals/100g – negligible (and 100g is a lot of mustard and cress).

Mustard and cress contains some protein and fibre, vitamin C, beta-carotene, folate and relatively small amounts of other vitamins and some minerals, but is usually eaten in small quantities.

Nectarine

An average fruit weighs about 120g and has 48 calories.

Nectarines are slightly more nutritious than peaches. They contain plenty of vitamin C and potassium, and are a useful source of fibre as well. They also have some beta-carotene and phytonutrients, and make good smoothies when mixed with some berries.

Nettles

see DANDELIONS AND WILD LEAVES

Noodles

Egg noodles have 391 cals/100g raw weight; broad rice noodles, 371; rice thread noodles, 383 and Japanese soba noodles, 360.

Watch the quantities of noodles you use. Egg noodles are high in protein and contain some fibre, but only small amounts of vitamins and minerals once cooked. Rice noodles have some phosphorus and a little fibre. Soba noodles are a better option; they are made from buckwheat and contain more fibre but are also easy to use and versatile. You may come across noodles made from mung beans – sometimes called cellophane noodles – which are digested comparatively slowly and have a low GI.

Nuts

see ALMONDS, BRAZIL NUTS, CASHEW NUTS, CHESTNUTS, COCONUTS, HAZELNUTS, MACADAMIA NUTS, PECANS, PEANUTS, PINE NUTS, PISTACHIOS, WALNUTS

Oatcakes

Allow an average of 55 calories per oatcake.

Oatcakes are a better option than most other crackers because they have some benefits from the oats they contain – fibre, most significantly – as well as some minerals and B vitamins. There are two potential problems, though: they may be high in salt, and they may contain palm oil, which is high in saturates. Go for ones made with olive oil instead.

Oatmeal

375 cals/100g.

Oats are high in fibre, particularly a form of soluble fibre called beta-glucan which has been shown to help lower the level of cholesterol circulating in the blood. They also contain B vitamins, have useful amounts of calcium, iron, magnesium and zinc and have more protein than most other grains. They are low GI, because of the fibre. Add them to bread or baking – or have porridge for breakfast.

see also PORRIDGE

Offal

Lamb's kidneys, fried, 188 cals/100g; calf's liver, fried, 176; chicken's liver, fried, 169; lamb's liver, fried, 237; stewed oxtail, 243; tripe, raw weight, 33.

Almost all offal is high in nutrients, and liver is especially high in vitamin A. In fact, it has so much that the official advice is to eat it in moderation, and not at all in early pregnancy. It's also one of the best sources of iron. All organ meat is high in B vitamins and has a range of minerals. Oxtail is higher in fat, and tripe has few real benefits apart from some protein and traces of vitamins; it's largely water.

Oils

All oils have essentially the same calories per 100ml: 899. There is a little variation across some brands, but work on this basis: a tablespoon is 135 calories and a teaspoon contains 45.

The types of oil vary in the benefits (or otherwise) they can bring – see pages 35–6 – so make wise choices. Generally go for olive or rapeseed oil, and avoid coconut and palm oil. Always measure oil; it's easy to pour more than you think. The quantities specified in most recipes can often be substantially reduced, so try that too.

Okra

Raw weight, 31 cals/100g. Boiled, they go down to 28, but deep-fry them and they rocket up to 269.

Okra is very high in fibre, particularly soluble fibre. It's got a lot of beta-carotene, useful amounts of manganese and potassium, and some vitamin C. Unlike some vegetables, it retains a lot of its nutrients when boiled.

Olives

Allow 5 calories per stuffed olive and 3 per unstuffed one.

Olives are a great snack for dieters – just watch the overall quantity. They are a good source of vitamin E and have plenty of antioxidants. Olives in brine can have high levels of salt, so drain and rinse them thoroughly. Some of the olive marinade mixtures available can also be quite high in calories – particularly those with cheese or lots of flavoured oil (and the oil often isn't olive oil) – so make your own.

....

Onions

Raw weight, 36 cals/100g; shallots have 20 cals/100g. Frying onions whacks up the count – 100g of fried onions contains 146 calories.

Onions contain antioxidants that have multiple benefits: they seem to boost the immune system, work like antibiotics in part and may even prevent the growth of cancer cells. The one thing to be aware of, though, is that cooking onions can add a lot of calories, so be careful and only use small amounts of oil. Try them raw, finely sliced in salads.

For pickled onions, see CHUTNEYS AND PICKLES

....

Oranges, etc.

Oranges, 37 cals/100g, weighed without the peel, and 60 for a medium fruit. Tangerines have 35 cals/100g and are 25 for a medium one; satsumas, 36 cals/100g and 25 for a medium one; clementines, 37 cals/100g, and a medium clementine is 25.

Oranges are a great source of vitamin C – citrus fruits are the most concentrated source of this vitamin – but also of thiamin and folate. The fine membrane between the segments is high in pectin, a soluble fibre, so it's better to eat the fruit rather than drink the juice. They're also high in antioxidant bioflavonoids. The smaller fruits like tangerines have proportionately lower levels of the nutrients, but still make an excellent contribution.

see also FRUIT AND VEGETABLE JUICE

....

Oxtail

see OFFAL

....

Oysters

Each, 18 calories.

Oysters are a great source of vitamin B12 and zinc, and have useful amounts of vitamin E, niacin, iron and potassium. They also contain some thiamin, riboflavin, selenium and iodine. They do contain cholesterol, like other shellfish, but this has little effect on the level of cholesterol in the blood.

Papaya

Fresh, 36 cals/100g; tinned in juice, 65.

Half a papaya contains the full recommended daily amount of vitamin C and is also extremely high in beta-carotene. Papayas are also very high in fibre – with good levels of soluble fibre – and have small amounts of calcium and iron. They also contain papain, an enzyme which helps digestion and has pain-relieving qualities. Squeeze on a little lime juice to enhance the flavour.

Parmesan

see CHEESE

Parsley

see HERBS

Parsnip

64 cals/100g.

A very useful source of fibre, parsnips also contain significant amounts of vitamins C and E, potassium, phosphorus and iron. They have vitamin B1, niacin, folate and beta-carotene. Just be careful not to add lots of fat when cooking them.

Passion fruit

36 cals/100g. A medium one will yield 35g of seeds and pulp – 13 calories.

A single passion fruit is very high in beta-carotene, as well as being a good source of vitamin C. They're also a great source of fibre.

Pasta

White pasta averages 345 cals/100g and wholemeal has 325; 100g dry weight is a good helping. Filled pastas can be significantly higher in calories, especially if they contain cheese, so check the packaging information.

Wholemeal pasta is a good source of fibre and niacin, and generally has a low GI. It also has twice the iron of white and more nutrients all round – and it's not as heavy as it used to be. White pasta has two thirds less fibre and is usually classed as medium GI. Always cook pasta lightly, so it still has some bite to it, and choose sauces carefully. Check the contents of any filled pasta and bear in mind that they are usually served with a sauce of some kind too – often melted butter. Try also to pass on the Parmesan.

Pasta sauces

Bought sauces can range from about 50 calories per 100ml to three times that, so check labels on individual brands.

Make your own, but avoid adding high-calorie ingredients like cream. When eating out, tomato-based sauces are the best choice; steer clear of those with lots of cheese, butter, cream or fatty meat. *See also* COOKING SAUCES

Pastry

Filo pastry has 234 cals/100g, raw weight, but you tend to add a lot of butter when you use it, though you can substitute a little olive or rapeseed oil instead. Flaky pastry, raw weight, has 427 cals/100g; puff pastry, 400; shortcrust, 451; wholemeal, 433.

Not only is pastry high in fat, it's high in saturated fat. Worth avoiding if you can!

Pâté

Check packaging here – a likely portion size is 50g. As a generalisation, the average liver pâté has 348 cals/100g, farmhouse, 367 and pâté de campagne, 300.

Pâtés are generally high in fat, but they often have surprisingly high levels of monounsaturated fats. They also contain good quantities of B vitamins (and liver pâtés are high in vitamin A) and iron, though, so don't rule them out completely. If they come with a layer of melted butter on top, remove it; never eat pâté with buttered bread or crackers but have them plain and watch portion sizes. If you do all that, you should still be able to enjoy pâté in moderation.

....

Pawpaw

see PAPAYA

....

Peaches

The average fruit weighs about 120g and has 40 calories.

Peaches are a good source of vitamin C (though they have slightly less than nectarines) and also contain some beta-carotene. Tinned peaches lose over 80 per cent of their vitamin C content, and are often canned in syrup – higher in calories.

....

Pecans

689 cals/100g.

Pecans are very high in fat, but a high proportion of that is monounsaturated. They are also rich in polyunsaturates and a good source of vitamin E and some minerals.

....

Peanut butter

A level teaspoon of smooth peanut butter has 30 calories, but do be careful – there are over 600 calories in 100g.

Some peanut butter contains palm oil, which is worth avoiding if you can, so read the ingredient lists for different brands. It is high in fat, like peanuts themselves, but also in monounsaturates (providing there's no palm oil). Peanut butter contains a good range of minerals and vitamins in useful quantities as well as high levels of niacin.

....

Peanuts

Plain, 563 cals/100g; dry roasted, 589; roasted, 602.

Peanuts aren't actually nuts. They're legumes, related to peas and beans, and grow underground, giving them their alternative name of groundnuts. They are, however, especially rich in essential fatty acids, like walnuts and hazelnuts, and are a great source of B vitamins, vitamin E and a range of minerals. Dry-roasted peanuts lose almost 90 per cent of their vitamin E; roasted and salted ones have even less. They both have about half the folate content. They are also high in salt, of course – the dry-roasted versions too.

Pears

64 calories for an average fruit, weighing 160g. They have 40 cals per 100g.

Pears are a good source of fibre (including soluble fibre – pectin), vitamin C, potassium and bioflavonoids. Like apples and bananas, they make a convenient snack to carry with you.

Peas

83 cals/100g raw; petits pois, 49; mushy peas, 81.

Peas are a great source of many vitamins and minerals as well as protein. They are a rich source of thiamin and have significant amounts of folate and phosphorus, but mangetout have more vitamin C. Frozen peas are perfectly good; they are actually more nutritious than fresh peas which have been sitting around after picking. Some of the vitamins are lost in boiling, though.

Peppers

The average pepper weighs 100g. Green ones have 15 calories each; yellow, 28; red or orange ones, 32.

Peppers are one of the best vegetable sources of vitamin C – weight for weight, they have more than twice that of oranges. They are also good for fibre and both beta-carotene – the precursor of vitamin A – and bioflavonoids. Red, orange and yellow peppers are riper than green ones. They have more sugars and often higher levels of nutrients, particularly red peppers which are massively richer in beta-carotene.

Persimmon

see SHARON FRUIT

Pesto

Bottled brands vary; they are about 440 cals/100g or 66 for a level tablespoon.

Home-made pesto is full of good things – pine nuts, raw garlic, olive oil as well as basil and Parmesan – but commercial versions may not contain them or use substitutes that are not as nutritionally valuable. They may also have preservatives and artificial colours. Try making your own; it isn't difficult (see page 79).

Pheasant

see GAME

Pickles

see CHUTNEY AND PICKLES

Pies

Fruit pies vary from about 185 cals/100g (for a wholemeal pie with just a top crust) to 356 cals/100g for individual ones, so check before you buy. A cheese and egg quiche is about 315 cals/100g.

Pastry is so high in calories that it's well worth restricting pies and quiches. They have all the problems of pastry, with added calories from the fillings. These may provide some nutrients, but there are better ways to get them when you're trying to lose weight.

see also CORNISH PASTY

Pigeon

see GAME

Pilchards

Canned in tomato sauce, pilchards have 144 cals/100g on average. One large pilchard is about 50g.

Pilchards are adult sardines. They are high in protein and great for monounsaturated fats and essential fatty acids, including omega 3. They are also an excellent source of vitamins D and E, as well as a useful way of getting B vitamins, especially B12. They're high in calcium as their fine bones are eaten, as well as in potassium, selenium and iodine. The tomato sauce provides lycopene.

see also TOMATOES

Pine nuts

688 cals/100g; and 70 for two heaped teaspoons.

Pine nuts are actually the edible seeds of a type of pine rather than true nuts, and are high in mono-and polyunsaturated fats. They also have a good range of minerals and are high in vitamin E and niacin. Make the most of them by adding them to salads or making your own pesto.

Pineapple

Fresh, 41 cals/100g; tinned in juice, 47; tinned in syrup, 64.

Pineapple is a useful source of vitamin C, but has few other vitamins or minerals. It does, however, contain bromelain, a phytochemical that breaks down proteins. This aids digestion as well as providing other benefits.

Pistachios

601 cals/100g for the kernels. Ten nuts, shelled, have 30 calories.

Pistachio nuts provide protein and fibre, and are particularly rich in potassium. They have good levels of calcium and also contain the B vitamins, especially folate and vitamin E and a range of minerals. Roasted pistachios can be quite salty.

Pizza

These are very, very variable, so check packaging if possible – a 20cm (8-inch) Margarita pizza with a thin base is, on average, 500 calories.

In restaurants, avoid ones with deep bases, lots of high-calorie toppings (like pepperoni or more cheese than usual), or anything extra large. The nutritional value of pizza depends on the topping: for instance, a cheese and tomato one would have protein, vitamin E, phosphorus, calcium and lycopene from the tomatoes, among other things. A wholemeal base – if at all possible – would add fibre.

Plaice

Raw weight, 79 cals/100g. Fried in breadcrumbs, it goes up to 228 cals/100g – in batter, up to 257 cals/100g. Fried plaice goujons have 426.

Like all white fish, plaice is a good source of protein with low levels of fat, but that can be changed by the way it is cooked – grilling is best and sauces are to be avoided. Plaice is good for vitamin B12, has smaller quantities of other B vitamins and also a range of minerals.

Plantain

Boiled, 112 cals/100g; fried, 267.

Plantains are sometimes called 'green bananas', but they are starchier than bananas and must be cooked. They are a source of vitamins A, B6, C and folate, as well as potassium and magnesium. They are a mainstay of West Indian cooking.

Plums

Fresh plums have 36 cals/100g – the weight of a large one. Damsons and greengages are about the same, but with smaller individual fruits; a greengage would be about 20 calories. Prunes (dried plums) are 141 cals/100g for the ready-to-eat version. Tinned prunes are 79 cals/100g in juice and 90 in syrup.

Fresh damsons, greengages and plums are good sources of fibre and potassium. Plums are not particularly high in vitamin C but also contain some vitamin E; the red and purple varieties are useful for the beta-carotene they contain. Prunes have more fibre and potassium and iron in useful quantities.

Polenta

Dry weight, 398 cals/100g. Ready-made polenta has about 70 calories for the same weight.

Polenta is coarsely ground cornmeal, mostly starchy carbohydrate and low in fibre. It is, however, gluten free, so it is useful for those who are gluten-intolerant. It contains potassium, iron, phosphorus and the B vitamin thiamin.

Pomegranate

About 70 calories for a medium fruit.

Pomegranates are a rich source of vitamin C and a great source of dietary fibre – to get the full benefits, eat the seeds rather than drinking the juice. You don't have to pick them out painstakingly with a pin, though. Cut the pomegranate in two, squeeze each half slightly then hold it upside down over a bowl and whack the skin with a wooden spoon. Most of the seeds will fall out.

Popadoms

see CRISPS AND SAVOURY SNACKS

Popcorn

Plain, 593 cals/100g; sweet, 480 (you get fewer sweet popcorn kernels to 100g).

High in fat, high in salt and/or sugar, not many nutritional benefits apart from some vitamin E – so keep popcorn for treats. Avoid extra-large mega portions if you're trying to lose weight.

Poppy seeds

560 cals/100g, but nobody uses this quantity normally. Half a teaspoon is more likely – 11 calories.

Nutritionally, the quantities of poppy seeds used are so small that any contribution is minimal, but do add them to stir-fries and salads for a bit of variety.

Pork

Average meat, trimmed of fat, raw weight: 123 cals/100g. Pork crackling is 548 – so resist if you can. Chops, raw weight, 270 cals/100g.

Pork is not actually the fatty meat it is often thought to be – there are some fatty cuts like belly pork, but generally lean pork is lower in fat than either beef or lamb. Trim visible fat, avoid those fatty cuts, and there is no reason to stop eating it. It's a great source of protein and B vitamins, and is also good for providing selenium, zinc and iron.

But no crackling! Many believe that it's a good idea to buy organic pork as pigs are routinely fed many drugs that remain in their meat.

....

Porridge

30g, dry weight, is enough for one person – approximately 110 calories.

Oats are fantastically healthy, a great source of soluble fibre. Quick-cook porridge is partially processed and lower in nutrients; ordinary porridge is actually quite quick to use anyway. It is low GI, providing a steady release of energy, and will keep you feeling full for longer. If you make porridge with milk measure the quantity you use; it will give more nutrients but also more calories – so don't forget to add them in. Try using chopped dried fruits instead of sugar or jam.

see also OATMEAL

....

Port

A 50ml pub measure contains 79 calories.

At 157 cals/100 ml, port is much more calorific than wine. It does have some minerals and possibly useful antioxidants but not in quantities that will make a difference.

see also WINE

....

Potatoes

New potatoes, raw weight, 70 cals/100g; old ones, 75. Watching cooking methods is essential: 100g of boiled new potatoes has 75 calories; the same quantity of baked potato – including the skin, a great fibre source – has 136; roast potatoes have 146. Old potatoes mashed with a small quantity of butter are 104. Chips, when home-made and fried, are 189 cals/100g, but 100g of chip-shop chips (only about 10 large ones) are 239 and may well be cooked in unhealthy fats. French fries from fast-food shops average at 280 or 364 if fine cut. Check the packaging information carefully on oven chips.

Potatoes cannot be included as part of the five-a-day count of fruit and vegetables, largely because of their high starch content. However, that doesn't mean they are bad; they can still be a useful source of vitamin C and fibre. The main problem lies in how they are cooked and eaten: in what oil or fat (lard, for instance, pushes up both calories and saturated fat), whether the skins are eaten or not, and whether anything fattening is served on them, like melting butter. Potatoes can easily be included in a weight-loss diet, and many people would be unhappy if they had to cut them out completely as some GI diets recommend, but be wise and watch quantities.

Prawns, shrimps and scampi

Boiled prawns have 99 cals/100g. Tiger prawns, with their shells, have 80 cals/100g and frozen shrimps, 73. They are generally a good choice when eating out, but beware of fried, breaded scampi – they have 237 cals/100g.

Plainly cooked and served, prawns and their close relatives are a great source of low-fat and low-calorie protein, but do be careful about cooking methods and any accompaniments like mayonnaise. They are all useful sources of vitamin B12; prawns contain significant quantities of selenium and iodine. Shrimps are great for iodine, have good levels of selenium and some calcium. All are high in cholesterol, but that shouldn't stop you eating them – cholesterol in the diet doesn't necessarily affect the level of cholesterol in the blood.

Prunes

see PLUMS

Puddings

The range of puddings available is enormous, and many are high in calories. Christmas pudding, for example, has 329 cals/100g and the average fruit crumble has 219.

When buying puddings in a shop check the calorie content listed on the packaging (and remember to see if the portion size looks realistic) and measure ingredients carefully if you are doing the cooking. To inspire you, remember that many ready-to-eat puddings have added artificial ingredients, colourings and preservatives. Fresh fruit is an excellent choice, but watch out for high-sugar syrups in fruit salads.

see also ICE CREAM AND FROZEN DESSERTS

Pulses

see BEANS, CHICKPEAS, LENTILS

Pumpkins and squashes

Pumpkin is 13 cals/100g raw weight; butternut squash is 36.

The orange-fleshed varieties are a good source of beta-carotene, vitamins C and E. They also contain phytoene (a carotenoid with possible anti-cancer properties) and a range of useful minerals. Watch cooking methods and don't forget to add the calories for any oil you might roast them with.

Pumpkin seeds

569 cals/100g; a level tablespoon has 85.

Seeds are very nutritious. Like other edible ones, pumpkin seeds are a great source of monounsaturated and polyunsaturated fats, and are also rich in potassium, iron, zinc, phosphorus and magnesium. Toast them in a dry frying pan and sprinkle them on salads.

Quiche

see PIES

Quinoa

Dry weight, 325 cals/100g.

A South American gluten-free grain, quinoa is a complete protein – very, very unusual in plants. It's also a useful source of some B vitamins, iron, potassium, magnesium, phosphorus and zinc, but isn't a brilliant source of fibre. It can be added to other grains and is a good addition to pilaffs or used as a nutty-tasting alternative to rice or pasta. It is low in fat and most of the oil it contains is monounsaturated.

Quorn

92 cals/100g.

Quorn is a product made from mycoprotein (a fungi) which is often used to make meat-free alternatives for food like sausages or stews. The calories vary for all the prepared food in which it is used, so check packs. It's a source of good-quality protein, fibre, zinc and magnesium, and is low in fat.

Rabbit

see GAME

Radishes

12 cals/100g.

Radishes are one of the Cruciferae and are a source of vitamin C. They're low in calories and fat – but don't dip them in lots of salt.

Raisins

see SULTANAS, CURRANTS AND RAISINS

Raspberries

25 cals/100g, which is a large helping.

All berries are fantastic for dieters. Raspberries are a good source of fibre and vitamin C and also contain useful amounts of vitamin E, folate, calcium, magnesium, potassium and iron.

Red mullet

Raw weight, 124 cals/100g.

Mullet is a high-protein fish with delicate flesh, which doesn't need lots of sauce to enhance its taste. It has plenty of vitamins B6, B12 and niacin, as well as a good range of minerals.

Rhubarb

Raw weight, 7 cals/100g.

Rhubarb is a good source of potassium, and contains vitamin C and manganese. It also contains oxalic acid (so don't eat the leaves and don't cook it in an aluminium pan) and this inhibits the absorption of calcium and iron. It's not particularly high in fibre. Watch the amount of sugar you use when cooking rhubarb and don't forget to add that to your calculation.

Rice

Calories by 100g dry weight: Basmati, 356; brown rice, 357; white rice, 359; average risotto rice, 350; wild rice, 347. A serving is often estimated at 75g dry weight, but 50g may well be enough. Allow 30 calories per tablespoon of boiled white rice.

The nutritional pluses (and minuses) of rice vary according to the type. All contain protein, carbohydrates and fibre, but most of the nutrients are found in the bran and the germ, and are either much reduced or absent in refined or processed rice. The GI is a good guide. Basmati rice has a lower GI than others because it contains more amylose – a starch which is digested quite slowly. Brown rice has more fibre and is a good complex carb, also lower GI; it has better levels of B vitamins than its white equivalent. Easy-cook rice is partly processed and will cause a swifter rise in blood sugar, leading more quickly to hunger – high GI. A lot of the starches in risotto rice break down during cooking rather than in the body, leading to a higher GI there too. Wild rice is, strictly speaking, not rice at all. It's a grass, and has twice the protein of white rice. It's also a good source of fibre and B vitamins, except B12.

Rice cakes

The average rice cake weighs 10g and contains 37 calories, but they do vary – check.

Some people like to use these as an alternative to crackers, but they are low in fibre and nutritional benefits. You'd be better with a low-salt oatcake made with olive oil.

Rocket

20 cals/100g, which would be a huge quantity – the calories are effectively negligible in a normal serving.

The nutritional benefits from a typical serving are similarly small, though vitamin C is at useful levels. Rocket is a peppery addition to a bowl of salad leaves.

Runner beans

22 cals/100g, raw weight.

Try small, young runner beans raw for the full range of nutritional goodies: beta-carotene, folate, vitamin C, fibre, potassium, iron – all in good quantities. About a third of their nutritional content is lost when they are boiled.

Salad dressings

This is another area with a lot of variation, so read labels carefully. These are by 100ml: blue cheese dressing, 457; Caesar, 335; French, 462; salad cream, 348; thousand island, 323.

Definitely a danger area, as these are so high in calories (and are very easy to overdo). It's best to make your own and control the contents; check ingredient lists on commercial brands, keeping an eye out for lots of preservatives and artificial ingredients. Adding cheese to a dressing immediately boosts its calorie content, so automatically avoid those.

see also MAYONNAISE

Salad leaves

see LETTUCE AND SALAD LEAVES, WATERCRESS, ROCKET

Salads, ready-made

Coleslaw made with mayonnaise has an average of 260 cals/100g; reduced-calorie versions are 67. Potato salad with mayo has 287 and rice salad, 165. By contrast, a bowl of green salad (60g) has about 7.

Do think about making your own rather than buying prepared salads like these. Many commercial varieties come at a high calorie cost and may contain ingredients without the best nutritional values, as well as colourings and preservatives.

see also LETTUCES AND SALAD LEAVES

Salami

see MEATS, COLD AND DELI

Salmon

Raw weight, 180 cals/100g; smoked salmon, 142.

An oily fish, salmon is a great source of monounsaturated fat and omega-3 polyunsaturates. It also has good levels of B vitamins, particularly niacin, vitamins D and E, potassium, phosphorus, selenium and iodine. The amount of omega 3 can vary according to what the fish have been feeding on, and is highest in wild salmon. Smoked salmon is also great for dieters, but has high levels of salt.

Sardines

Canned in brine, 172 cals/100g; canned in oil (and drained), 220; canned in tomato sauce, 162. Fresh sardines have 198 cals/100g.

Sardines are young pilchards, and like them are high in omega 3s. They're a good source of iron and zinc, as well as other minerals, B vitamins and vitamin D. Tinned ones are great for calcium as the bones are eaten; choose those canned in tomato sauce as it contains lycopene, a valuable antioxidant. Fresh sardines are usually grilled and are delicious when barbecued.

Sauces, table

These are mostly used in moderation, so the calorie figures given are by the level tablespoon: barbecue, 14; brown, 15; horseradish, 23; mint, 15; tartare, 45, Worcestershire sauce, 10. Thai fish sauce has 22.

They don't make a big nutritional contribution overall, but watch sugar and salt content – and quantity.

see also TOMATO KETCHUP, SOY SAUCE

Sauerkraut

Drained, 9 cals/100g.

The flavour of this pickled cabbage comes from fermentation, and the fermentation bacteria may help the growth of 'good' bacteria in the gut. It's also a good source of vitamin C.

Sausages

Here are some average figures – read packaging, too. Pork sausages, raw weight, 309 cals/100g; beef, 286. Sausage rolls are about 383 cals/100g and are best avoided. Black pudding has 297 cals/100g; white pudding, 450; boiled haggis has 310.

All sausages can be very high in fat – saturated fat – and in salt. They may contain lots of additives, too. In general, they have the same nutritional qualities as fresh meat but in lower quantities, so go for those with the most meat to get the most benefits. Black pudding is also high in iron. Cook sausages so that they can shed fat rather than gain it, so grill or bake them on a rack; dry-frying is the next best choice. Never add more fat.

see also MEATS, COLD AND DELI

....

Savoury snacks

see CRISPS AND SAVOURY SNACKS

....

Scallops

118 cals/100g.

Scallops are high in vitamin B12 and niacin, potassium, phosphorus and selenium; they also have useful amounts of zinc and iodine. They are lower in cholesterol than some other forms of seafood, not that this has an effect on blood cholesterol to any great extent.

....

Scampi

see PRAWNS, SHRIMPS AND SCAMPI

....

Scotch eggs

They do vary in weight, but average 240 cals/100g.

Sausage meat wrapped round an egg and then fried – hmm. Not a good idea. Even the smaller ones which are filled with minced egg are high in calories and fat. Worth giving up or severely restricting.

....

Sea bass

112 cals/100g raw weight.

Sea bass is usually plainly cooked to preserve its taste, and is an excellent choice though it can be expensive. It's high in protein, low in calories and contains good amounts of vitamin B12 and the minerals calcium, iron and phosphorus.

Seaweeds

Nori has 303 cals/100g; wakame, 93 cals/100g; kombu has 63. In all cases you'd be unlikely to use more than 10g – a whole pack of nori is only 25g, and a single sheet weighs about 2g.

Edible seaweeds are rich in iodine, high in potassium and calcium, as well as a range of other minerals. Many are good sources of B vitamins and beta-carotene as well. Unusually for plants, they contain significant amounts of vitamin B12, but it may not be in a useful form; research continues. Seaweeds, however, are often quite high in salt. Most of the Japanese ones can be found in health-food shops, and even in supermarkets, but local varieties are worth tracking down too. Laver (same seaweed as nori) is high in protein and a range of vitamins as well as iodine. Dulse is rich in potassium and magnesium, and carragheen in vitamin A and the B vitamins.

Sesame seeds

598 cals/100g; a teaspoon has 30.

Like other seeds, sesame seeds are very nutritious. They are a good source of protein and calcium, iron, vitamin E and niacin. Toast them in a dry frying pan and sprinkle them on stir-fried vegetables.

Shallots

see ONIONS

Sharon fruit and persimmons

80 cals/100g, a medium fruit.

These are a great source of bioflavonoids, polyphenols which can help metabolise fat. They are also high in beta-carotene, potassium, calcium and iron. Unripe persimmons are unpalatable, but Sharon fruit have been bred to be acceptable when hard.

Shellfish

see COCKLES, CRAB, LOBSTER, MUSSELS, OYSTERS; PRAWNS, SHRIMPS
AND SCAMPI; SCALLOPS; WHELKS AND WINKLES

Sherry

*Per 50ml bar measure, dry and medium sherries have 58 calories,
while sweet sherry has 68.*
Be careful about the size of your measure – errors can make a big
difference to calories.

Skate

72 cals/100g, raw weight.
Skate is a cartilaginous fish, like shark. They are generally low in fat
but must be eaten fresh. Skate is often served with a butter sauce
which is worth avoiding. As with all fish, the protein content is
excellent and skate has a good range of B vitamins, iodine and
phosphorus.

Smoked fish

The distinct flavour of smoked fish should come from the naturally
occurring chemicals in smoke and not from a test tube, but this is
not always the case.It is worth buying the best you can because
cheaper smoked fish is often artificially dyed; naturally smoked fish
is not bright orange or lurid yellow but gets its colour from the
smoking process. The chemicals in the smoke also help to prevent
the growth of bacteria and give a specific taste and, yes, some of
them are carcinogenic – but only in large quantities. The associated
risks are much, much lower than those connected to tobacco smoke.
In addition, the modern fashion is for a light smoke. There really is
no need to be concerned unless you eat a lot of smoked food on a
regular basis.

Smoothies

see FRUIT SMOOTHIES

Soups

Both shop-bought and home-made soups vary enormously in nutritional content, but they are a great part of any weight-loss diet. Check calorie counts on packaging – even the most apparently healthy soups can be high – and make sensible choices. The canning process affects nutrients, and many commercial soups include ingredients you'd be unlikely to encounter in the average kitchen. Avoid anything with high-calorie ingredients like cream, and don't use lots of oil to pre-fry the ingredients if you are making soup at home. If you use water or a home-made vegetable stock, you can keep salt to a minimum. Making your own soup is also a good way to add pulses to your diet.

Soy sauce, shoyu and tamari

Soy sauce has 6 calories per tablespoon; shoyu, 13 and tamari, 20.
Soy sauce is often high in salt and may have added caramel, but it is not generally used in large quantities.

Soya milk

Sweetened soya milk with calcium has 43 cals/100ml; unsweetened has 26 and 'light' unsweetened has 21.
Soya milk is ideal for people with lactose intolerance, as well as for those who prefer not to use animal products. It's high in protein, but isn't a good source of calcium or vitamin B12, unlike milk. Always choose soya milk that has been fortified with calcium if your intake is likely to be low and check soya 'cream' – some brands are very sugary. Many studies have shown beneficial effects from consuming soya protein, but you do need a lot for it to have a significant effect.
see also TOFU AND TEMPEH

Spices

Use these freely: they won't make a difference in terms of calories, but they will in terms of taste and flavour, so go for it. You won't need as much salt in dishes if you use spices.

Spinach

Raw, 25 cals/100g; boiled, 19.

Popeye was right – or nearly. Spinach is a wonderful source of nutrients, but it's not as high in iron as people used to think (that misconception apparently arose from a misplaced decimal point). It's a good source of beta-carotene and the carotenoid lutein, both of which are antioxidants, and it's high in vitamin K and folate. It does contain oxalic acid, like rhubarb, which hinders the absorption of calcium and iron. Raw baby spinach leaves are a delicious addition to salads. Always cook spinach in the bare minimum of water to preserve as many nutrients as possible; in fact, all you need is the water that clings to the leaves after they've been rinsed.

Spirits

All spirits – brandy, gin, rum, whisky and vodka – have 56 calories to a 25ml bar measure.

This measure isn't much and most people pouring spirits are likely to serve substantially more. Buy a pub measure and test it out; you may be surprised. Watch mixers, too, as they can add a lot of calories.

Spreads and margarines

There's huge calorie variation with these, so check packaging: very low-fat spreads can have only 183 cals/100g, while others can have as many as 645.

Most packs give some idea of how many you can expect in an average helping – 5g is enough to lightly cover a large slice of toast. There are health issues to consider too; avoid anything with high levels of hydrogenated fats (see page 35).

Spring greens

33 cals/100g, raw.

Another member of the crucifer family, like broccoli, cabbage and kale, spring greens have great nutritional benefits. They have similar phytochemicals to kale, but lots more calcium, niacin, vitamin C and beta-carotene. Kale is higher in folate, though.

Spring onions

6 calories to five trimmed spring onions.

The green parts of the stalks contain beta-carotene and folate, though spring onions are not usually eaten in quantities that make a nutritional difference. They have some of the same properties as onions.

....

Squashes

see PUMPKINS AND SQUASHES

....

Squid

70 cals/100g, raw weight.

Avoid any squid which is covered in breadcrumbs, batter or deep-fried – the extra calories can be substantial. Squid contains some B vitamins (especially niacin) and vitamin E, as well as a good selection of minerals. It is also very high in cholesterol, but this should not cause problems for most people.

....

Stilton

see CHEESE

....

Stock cubes

Most cubes average about 240 cals/100g, but you wouldn't use anything near that much.

These concentrated essences of meat or vegetables are often high in salt – one cube can have the equivalent of a whole teaspoon of salt. It's worth checking the other ingredients too, as you may find MSG or lots of sugar in some.

....

Strawberries

Fresh, 27 cals/100g.

Strawberries have higher levels of vitamin C than most other berries and, weight for weight, more than oranges. They are also a great source of fibre, folate and antioxidants which some experts think block the action of cancer cells.

Suet

Avoid this if you can. Ordinary suet is 826 cals/100g; vegetarian suet is even higher at 836 calories and both are often high in saturates and trans fats.

Sugar

20 calories per teaspoon, and per cube. Fructose is an alternative; it has the same basic calories but is much sweeter – you use 60g where you would use 100g of sugar, for example.

Sugar gives almost instant energy, but that's the problem – see page 51. The boost you get doesn't last and it comes at a substantial calorie cost. The calories in sugar are often called 'empty calories' because they have no value in nutritional terms.

Sultanas, currants and raisins

Sultanas have 275 cals/100g; currants, 267 and raisins, 272.

These are good sources of potassium and iron and are useful for the fibre they contain. They are, however, a concentrated source of energy as they have a high natural sugar content – and that means calories. Watch the quantities, and avoid any coated ones – they really don't need chocolate too.

Sunflower seeds

581 cals/100g. A level tablespoon contains 87 calories.

Edible seeds have lots of nutritional virtues, with many minerals and good fats. Sunflower seeds have some fibre and are high in vitamin E. They are also a source of B vitamins and contain useful levels of linoleic acid, a fatty acid essential for maintaining cell membranes.

Swede and turnips

Swede has 24 cals/100g raw weight; turnips have 23.

Both swedes and turnips are a useful source of vitamin C and fibre. They also contain indoles, phytochemicals which may protect against the development of cancer (dandelion roots are another source of these). Cooking makes it easier for the body to absorb the nutrients they contain. They are members of the crucifers, like broccoli and cabbage. Turnip tops – the leaves – make a good vegetable, because they are a source of beta-carotene and folate.

Sweetcorn

Tinned baby corn has 23 cals/100g. Corn on the cob varies in weight, but is 111 cals/100g when cooked.

Sweetcorn is high in fibre and vitamin C and rich in starch. It also contains some beta-carotene, vitamin C and B vitamins. Canned sweetcorn can be salty, so rinse it well.

Sweeteners

A teaspoon of most artificial sweeteners contains either no calories or very few, but they may have unfortunate side effects (such as alarming laxative qualities). It's better to try and wean yourself off sweet tastes altogether.

Sweet potato

87 cals/100g, raw weight.

Sweet potatoes are often cited as a substitute for ordinary potatoes in GI diets. They contain less starch and more fibre, and therefore have a lower GI. Those with orange flesh are high in beta-carotene – white ones have much, much less – and contain vitamin C and potassium as well as small quantities of other minerals and vitamins.

Sweets

There are so many different ones available. Here are a few, per 100g: boiled sweets, 327; pastilles, 284; peppermints, 395; liquorice allsorts, 349; sherbet sweets, 355; toffees, 426. Read packaging and check pack sizes too – it's not always clear.

It really is best to avoid 'empty calories' like these – calories that bring few nutritional benefits other than a swift sugar high. They can have a bad effect on your health as well as your diet, so reduce them or cut them out.

see also CHOCOLATE

Swiss chard and leaf beet
20 cals/100g.
These are high in vitamins A and C, as well as calcium and potassium, but watch the cooking method you use and preserve those levels as much as possible.

....

Swordfish
Fillet, 124 cals/100g raw weight.
Swordfish contains reasonable levels of omega-3 fatty acids as well as niacin, vitamin B6, B12, selenium, potassium and phosphorus.

....

Syrups
Golden syrup has 45 calories per level tablespoon; treacle, 41; molasses, 49; maple syrup, 52.
Syrups are liquid sugar, basically, and have the same problems for anyone trying to eat more healthily – more empty calories. Molasses is a useful source of vitamin B6 and has more nutrients than others, but not enough to compensate for the disadvantages.

....

Tahini
634 cals/100g for light tahini; 678 for dark.
Tahini is sesame seed paste, with the benefits of sesame seeds. It is high in fat, but the fat is mostly mono- and polyunsaturated. It's also high in protein and in a range of minerals, including calcium. There are good levels of B vitamins and it's also a source of vitamin E.

....

Tangerines
see ORANGES ETC.

....

Taramasalata
see DIPS

....

Tea
There are no calories in black or herb tea – but if you add milk, sugar or honey it's a different story. Black tea contains quercetin (an

antioxidant bioflavanoid also found in, for example, apples) and the level of catechins in green tea may prevent cancer cells forming; they also seem to help protect artery walls. Tea is a gentle stimulant as it contains caffeine. Herb teas do not have caffeine – and they are also zero-calorie drinks.

Tofu and tempeh

62 cals/100g, uncooked. Steamed tofu is 73 cals/100g, but steamed and fried is 261. Tempeh is 150 cals/100g, uncooked. Try not to deep-fry it, but boil or steam it instead.

Both of these are made from soya beans, and lots of research has shown that eating more soya can have significant health advantages, so do experiment if you haven't used them before. Soya beans are complete proteins and contain a wealth of phytoestrogenes, isoflavones which have been linked to lower rates of heart disease and some types of cancer (they are the best source for these). They do contain fat, but very largely 'good' fats; tofu is a good source of omega 3. Tempeh is another soya product, often used in Indonesian cooking. It's also high in protein, potassium, calcium and zinc.

Tomato ketchup

115 cals/100ml – a level tablespoon has 18.

Just watch how much you use. Normally, quantities are small but tomato ketchup doesn't contribute a lot, nutritionally speaking. It does contain carotenoids, like tomatoes, but it is frequently high in sugar and salt.

Tomatoes

17 cals/100g, the weight of a large fresh tomato, but watch how you cook them: grilled, they're 20 cals/100g and fried tomatoes shoot up to 91. Canned tomatoes are 19 cals/100g and tomato purée is 76 cals/100ml – about 12 per tablespoon. Sun-dried tomatoes are 60 cals/100g, and it's worth avoiding the ones in oil – they are very difficult to drain thoroughly and are high in calories (usually over 450 cals/100g).

Tomatoes bring important benefits to any diet. They contain B vitamins, notably folate, and are high in antioxidants – beta-carotene, vitamins C and E and also lycopene. Lycopene is a carotenoid which has been shown to help protect from both cardio-vascular disease and cancer. It is much more potent when tomatoes are cooked (canned ones are a good source). It is also fat-soluble, so cook tomatoes with something like a little olive oil for the maximum effect. This combination is one of the mainstays of the ultra-healthy Mediterranean diet.

Tonic water
see MIXERS

Treacle
see SYRUPS

Tripe
see OFFAL

Trout
A whole trout averages 225g raw weight and has 220 calories. Grilled, it's 135 cals/100g.

Trout is an oily fish that belongs to the same family as salmon. It's a good source of protein and essential fatty acids; vitamin A; B vitamins, especially B12 and vitamin D. It also contains vitamin E and has useful levels of potassium, phosphorus, selenium and iodine.

Tsatsiki
see DIPS

Tuna
Tuna tinned in spring water has 79 cals/100g; in brine, 99 and in oil, 189. Fresh tuna steaks are 150 cals/100g.

Though tuna is classed as an oily fish, tinned tuna actually contains relatively little omega 3; a lot of the natural oils are lost in the canning process. Tuna in brine can be very salty and should always be rinsed, but it is much lower in fat than tuna canned in oil; spring water is the best option. It contains a good range of minerals, vitamin D, some vitamin E and B vitamins. Niacin levels are particularly high. Fresh tuna is a much better source of essential fatty acids and contains a similar range of vitamins and minerals.

Turkey

Raw weights: dark meat, 104 cals/100g; white, 105. Roasted, the dark meat is 177 and the white, 153.

Turkey is an excellent low-fat source of protein, lower in fat than chicken. A skinned turkey breast, for instance, is 8 per cent fat; a skinned chicken breast is 21 per cent fat. Turkey has excellent levels of B vitamins and is good for potassium and phosphorus, and fine for selenium. It contains more zinc and iron than chicken, particularly the dark meat – so don't avoid it. Do avoid eating the skin, though, as it is high in both calories and saturated fat. Like all meats, ready-made turkey products are often highly processed and contain a lot of additives.

Turnips

see SWEDE AND TURNIPS

Vegetables

see ARTICHOKES, ASPARAGUS, AUBERGINE, BEETROOT, BROCCOLI, BRUSSELS SPROUTS, CABBAGE, CARROTS, CASSAVA, CAULIFLOWER, CELERIAC, CELERY, CHICORY, CHINESE LEAVES, COURGETTE, ENDIVE, FENNEL, GREEN OR FRENCH BEANS, KALE, KOHLRABI, LEEKS, MANGETOUT, MOOLI, OKRA, ONIONS, PARSNIP, PEAS, PEPPERS, PLANTAIN, POTATOES, RADISHES, RUNNER BEANS, SPINACH, SPRING GREENS, SPRING ONIONS, SWEDES AND TURNIPS, SWEETCORN, SWEET POTATO, SWISS CHARD, WATERCRESS, YAM

Venison

see GAME

Vermouth

Per 50ml bar measure, dry vermouth has 55 calories while sweet vermouth has 74.

Vermouths are rarely served without mixers, so be careful about which you use as that can make a big difference to overall calorie content.

Vinegar

Balsamic vinegar has 15 calories per tablespoon; other vinegars have 3.

Vinegar can be freely used in salad dressings – just be more cautious with balsamic. Explore flavoured vinegars, as well; they can add a lot of taste.

Walnuts

688 cals/100g; allow 25 for half a large one.

Walnuts are especially rich in antioxidants, but do have slightly lower levels of vitamins and minerals than many other nuts. They are a great source of protein and are particularly rich in Omega 3 fatty acids, which can help to lower the risk of heart attack and stroke.

Water chestnuts

Canned, 31 cals/100g.

Water chestnuts provide low-calorie crunch in stir-fries, but very little else – they contain a small amount of protein and carbohydrate and an awful lot of water.

Watercress

22 cals/100g, without the thick stalks.

Another of the Cruciferae, like broccoli; watercress is one of the healthiest salad vegetables. It's high in antioxidants: a great source of beta-carotene and vitamin C as well as isothiocyanate, which appears to break down the elements in tobacco smoke that cause cancer. There are high levels of minerals and vitamins as well.

Watermelon

31 cals/100g.

Watermelon has a high GI but a low GL; though it does contain a lot of sugars (hence the high GI value), a normal portion isn't big enough to make a huge difference to your blood sugar level. Like all melons, it has a high water content. It has only traces of minerals – there is more potassium – but does contain useful levels of beta-carotene, though much less than canteloupe melon. It makes delicious juices and smoothies.

Wensleydale

see CHEESE

Whelks and winkles

Boiled whelks, 89 cals/100g; winkles, 72.

These are high in protein, like other shellfish, and low in fat. They are a source of B vitamins and some minerals and may also have high salt levels, depending on how they are cooked.

Whitebait

As these small fishes are coated in flour and deep fried, they are high: 525 cals/100g.

Like all oily fish, they contain valuable nutrients – and calcium, as you eat the bones – but the high cost in calories probably isn't worth it.

Wine

Watch glass sizes when enjoying wine. These figures are for 175ml: red, 119; dry white, 116; medium white, 130; rosé, 124; sparkling white, 130. There are 750ml in an average bottle.

Be careful with quantities, as with all alcohol. Pub measures are often 125ml, but bigger glasses of up to 250ml are more common in many wine bars and restaurants – and at home. Red wine may have some beneficial effects due to the phytochemicals the grapes contain.

Yam

114 cals/100g; 133 for boiled yam.

Yam is a good source of potassium and, in the case of yellow-fleshed ones, of beta-carotene. They are sometimes confused with sweet potatoes, but contain 50 per cent more protein.

Yoghurt drinks

On average, 50 calories for a small pot, but check individual brands; light versions are sometimes available.

These are sometimes high in sugar and are often sold as 'containing probiotic bacteria'. Be aware that there are, presently, no regulations covering these statements. Tests have shown that many which claimed to have probiotics didn't contain the ones listed on the packaging – and some had none whatsoever. Some did contain them but they were, effectively, dead: useless. Don't buy these because of any claims made for them, but they can be convenient to include in a packed lunch if you're happy about the level of sugar.

Yoghurts

Most non-diet yoghurt is about 1 calorie per gram, so a 125g pot has 125 calories. There are lots of variations with different additions, different levels of fat and across different brands, so check information on the pots carefully.

Yoghurt is a great source of protein and calcium and is relatively low in calories, even the full-fat versions. People who are lactose intolerant can often tolerate yoghurt, as much of the lactose has been altered by fermentation. Yoghurt contains riboflavin and vitamin B12; a whole-milk yoghurt has more calcium than a low-fat one; flavoured yoghurts have less. Low-fat yoghurts may have added sugar to compensate for the lack of taste, and may contain artificial sweeteners, flavourings and colours; otherwise, they are great for anyone's diet.

Further reading

Bodyfoods for Busy People, Jane Clarke, 2004

Eat, Drink and Be Healthy, Walter Willett, 2001

The Exercise Bible, Joanna Hall, 2003

Fat is a Feminist Issue, Susie Orbach, 1998

Fitness for Life, Matt Roberts, 2002

The Food Bible, Judith Wills, 2006

The GI Diet, Rick Gallop, 2004

L is for Label: How to read between the lines on food packaging, Amanda Ursell, 2004

Low Calorie Dieting for Dummies, Susan McQuillan, 2005

The Low GI Diet, Jenny Brand-Miller, Kaye Foster-Powell and Joanna McMillan-Price, 2004

Need to know? Calorie Counting, Kate Santon, 2007

Nutrition for Dummies, Nigel Denby, Sue Baic and Carol Ann Rinzler, 2005

Nutrition for Life, Lisa Hark and Darwin Deen, 2005

Vitamins and Minerals Handbook, Amanda Ursell et al., 2004

The Weight-Loss Bible, Joanna Hall, 2005

Workouts for Dummies, Tamilee Webb, 1998

There are some good books which explore the subject of children and diet in a very user-friendly way (they have much more helpful information too):

First-time Parent, Lucy Atkins, 2006 – good on how to feed babies and small children

From Kid to Superkid, Paul Sacher, 2005 – healthy eating for children from the age of five

Yummy, Jane Clarke, 2006 – excellent on all aspects of feeding children

Useful addresses

British Dietetic Association
5th Floor, Charles House,
148-9 Great Charles Street
Queensway
Birmingham, B3 3HT
www.bda.uk.com

British Nutrition Foundation
High Holborn House
52-54 High Holborn
London, WC1V 6RQ
www.nutrition.org.uk

Eating Disorders Association
1 Prince of Wales Rd
Norwich, NR1 1DW
www.edauk.com
Tel: 0845 634 1414 (adult
helpline);
0845 634 7650 (youth helpline)

The Vegetarian Society
Parkdale
Dunham Rd
Altrincham
Cheshire, WA14 4QG
www.vegsoc.org

Women's Health Concern
PO BOX 2126
Marlow,
Bucks, SL7 2RY
www.womens-health-concern.org

Index